Universal He

D0006271

Universal Health Care

What the United States Can Learn from the Canadian Experience

**PAT ARMSTRONG AND HUGH ARMSTRONG
WITH CLAUDIA FEGAN, M.D.**

THE NEW PRESS

NEW YORK

Library of Congress Cataloging-in-Publication Data

Armstrong, Pat, 1945–
    Universal Health Care: What the United States Can Learn from the Canadian
Experience /Pat Armstrong and Hugh Armstrong, with Claudia Fegan, M.D.
        108p.   cm.
    Includes bibliographical references.
    ISBN 1-56584-410-6
    1. National health insurance—Canada. 2. Medical care—Canada. I. Armstrong, Hugh,
1943–   II. Fegan, Claudia. III. Title
RA412.5.C3A76   1998
362.1'0971—dc21   97-41011

Published in the United States by The New Press, New York
Distributed by W. W. Norton & Company, Inc., New York

The New Press was established in 1990 as a not-for-profit alternative to the large,
commercial publishing houses currently dominating the book publishing industry.
The New Press operates in the public interest rather than for private gain,
and is committed to publishing, in innovative ways, works of educational, cultural, and
community value that might not be considered sufficiently profitable.
The New Press's editorial offices are located at the City University of New York.

Printed in the United States of America

9 8 7 6 5 4 3 2

Acknowledgments

All books have multiple and diverse origins. This book is no exception. But it can be directly traced to Leo Panitch. When this professor of political science and internationally recognized scholar was asked by André Schiffrin, Director of The New Press, about who could write a book on the Canadian health care system for an American audience, Leo recommended the Armstrongs.

Excited by such an assignment, the Armstrongs also felt hesitant about writing on health care for readers across the border. To address this concern, they sought an American collaborator who was knowledgeable about the health care systems in both the United States and Canada. Claudia Fegan, a Chicago physician and former president of Physicians for a National Health Program, generously responded to the Armstrongs' request for support. In Claudia, the Armstrongs found not only the expertise they sought but also an efficient and supportive collaborator who brought a fine sense of humor and proportion to the task.

For her part, Claudia would like to thank her office manager, Mike Spain, who tended to the little details necessary to make a long distance project such as this go. Thanks to Alan Sebastiani for keeping our Medicare facts correct. A special thanks to her twin brother, Billy Davis, who encouraged her. Most of all she wants to thank her husband, Dan, and her children, Angela and Jimmy, who are ever supportive of all her efforts to make a difference in health care.

For their part, the Armstrongs would like to thank Leo for his faith in their abilities. It is particularly important to have the support of such a principled man. Lyn Spink enthusiastically agreed to read a very messy manuscript and offered comments that were at once encouraging and usefully critical. It was important to the Armstrongs to have such a meticulous scholar assess their progress and provide an American-Canadian perspective on the text. Both Lyn and Laura Sky continued to be essential to the Armstrongs' sanity, at the same time as they provided solid information and sound political advice. Martha Livingston and Shelley O'Neill regularly produced documents that were necessary for the research but difficult to access. Susan Dallin and John Hollingsworth often went beyond the call of research assistance, with John in particular working through the night to finish some technical work. Floyd Hembruff provided, as always, the physical and social space needed to complete the work. And finally, the Armstrongs would once again like to thank their daughters Jill and Sarah. Jill and Sarah now form part of the Armstrong research team, doing everything from research to typing to tea. Without them, this book would not have reached the printer.

The New Press has been everything a publisher should be. It gently pushed for completion without harassment. André Schiffrin assisted by Jessica Blatt have kept in regular contact and have always been available to answer our questions. Matt Weiland supported us with kind comments and useful information. The copy-editing was both respectful and thorough, exactly what authors need.

And finally, we would like to thank all those on both sides of the border who have fought for, and continue to fight for, universal, accessible, comprehensive, portable and publicly administered health care.

Contents

List of Tables

Preface

American health care is at a crossroads. In the past fifty years, the profession of medicine has become the business of medicine, and many people are unhappy with the results. The mission to relieve pain and suffering has been supplanted by the drive to maximize profit and the cost has been tremendous. Along the way, innocence and idealism have been lost, trust has eroded, and health care professionals find themselves uncertain as to who they are to serve.

Patients agonize over managed care denials. Physicians lament the loss of control and try to figure out how medicine could have gone so wrong. Many in the United States look for solutions to the current health care crisis. However, before we can solve a problem we have to define it.

In the United States today, at any given time, there are more than forty-one million people who are without health insurance. This does not include the millions who are woefully underinsured, including the millions of women of child-bearing age whose health insurance does not cover prenatal benefits and families for whom a single hospitalization would mean economic catastrophe. A recent survey by the U.S. Census Bureau showed that in the previous three years, more than sixty million people had been uninsured for a month or more. Think about what it means to be uninsured.

Many of the uninsured are young, healthy people who do not think about their health on a daily basis or what it would mean to lose it.

There are those who may have health concerns, but fear a visit to a physician might mean a test they could never afford. There are those who have a family member who requires care which absorbs all of the assets of the household. There are those who, on a regular basis, must decide between a prescribed medication and household expenses, such as rent. There are millions of people who, on a daily basis, do not have access to health care in a country where physicians and hospitals are in abundance. Health care did not become a hot political issue in the United States until it became an economic issue.

In 1988, Lee Iacocca, then head of Chrysler, went before Congress to explain that he spent more on the health care benefits for the auto workers that build a car than on the steel that went into that car. Specifically, Chrysler spent $700 per car on the health benefits of the auto workers who built that car in Detroit. Chrysler could build the same car across the bridge in Windsor, Ontario, and spend only $223 (U.S.) on health benefits. This was the same auto workers union and the same level of benefits. Simply, the cost of health care benefits was stagnating the economy and inhibiting the ability of U.S. companies to compete on a global level.

As a consequence of these revelations, health care became a hot political issue in the 1992 election. In a special election held in November of 1991 to fill a prematurely vacated seat for the United States Senate from Pennsylvania, Harris Wofford (who had never run for political office) upset former Attorney General Dick Thornburgh. Thornburgh had been then President Bush's hand-picked candidate for that seat. Wofford's success focused the attention of the nation on the issue of health care. Harris Wofford said, "a Constitution that guaranteed the right to an attorney if you commit a crime should guarantee you the right to a physician if you get sick." He spoke to a need the public was feeling. The election of Harris Wofford changed the political landscape for the 1992 election. Suddenly, the Democratic Party was seen as sensitive to issues the Republicans were willing to ignore.

The Clinton Plan, which became the proposed solution to the health care crisis, relied on competition between large insurance companies to control costs. This was based on the belief that applying business principles, specifically market forces, to health care would finally bring health care costs under control (i.e., if there was competition for the costs of services, prices would come down). An example of how this does not work is a 1990 study which showed there were 10,000 mammography machines in the United States. It would have taken only 2000 machines to meet the needs of the women who were obtaining mammograms regularly. If all women got all of the recommended screening exams, only 5132 machines would be needed. Because there are too many machines, each exam costs more. Many mammographers perform too few exams to maintain their competence, thus the quality of the exams they perform suffer. Competition creates duplication of expensive technology in health care, not cost effectiveness.

Instead of finding a new solution, in the past five years we have watched more and more people come under the control of fewer and fewer companies. Many of these companies are for-profit insurance companies. There is not a comprehensive policy to provide for the health care needs of U.S. citizens. Health care dollars are not necessarily allocated on the basis of determinants of health such as the public health needs of a community, but, instead, on the basis of capital leverage. Those companies large enough to win the contracts from various employers win the right, not only to provide health care, but to limit access to health care as well. As insurers, they can determine what services will and will not be available to various segments of the population. These companies do not earn the right to determine access to care based on their ability to produce a comprehensive public health policy that will address the health needs and goals of the population they are serving. They earn this right based on their ability to provide service at the cheapest price. Large insurance companies compete not just for contracts to provide coverage for the employees of private firms, but to be the providers for recipients of public programs such as Medicaid and Medicare as well.

Winston Churchill once said, "You can count on Americans to do the right thing, but only after they have tried every thing else." We have tried to ignore the issue of the uninsured and the underinsured. We have looked for private solutions to the problem. We have begun to pay a price that is immeasurable. We pay not just in terms of care delayed, which is always more costly. We also pay in terms of a stagnant work force with decreased productivity. Thirty-five percent of people in the United States earning between $15,000 and $50,000 yearly stayed in an unwanted job to keep their health insurance. We can not expect large for-profit insurance companies to solve this problem. These companies' first responsibility is to their shareholders, not the public's health.

There is often talk about political feasibility in the United States when considering solutions to this problem. Solutions to the current health care crisis are often discarded before being considered or evaluated, because there are those who believe they are not politically feasible. Yet, we are a nation of individuals that has often battled the odds, a nation that cheers for the underdog, a nation born of a refusal to accept the status quo. How can we so quickly dismiss a solution to such a devastating problem because politicians tell us and insurance companies tell us it is not politically feasible? Perhaps there is something we have missed. *Universal Health Care* is the story of the Canadian solution and a challenge to the U.S. public.

The Canadians got it right! They provided health care for all Canadians with the Canada Health Act. Five basic principles, which any Canadian will proudly recite for you, form the basis for a comprehensive public health policy: public administration, comprehensiveness, universality, portability, and accessibility. Public administration avoids the profiteering and thus the additional 20–30% overhead and profit associated with for-profit companies. The overhead seen in the public sector is only a fraction of this.

Comprehensiveness means all necessary services are covered. Unless everything is covered potential savings are lost if patients delay preventive care or necessary care due to financial concerns, to say nothing of the human cost of care delayed.

Universality means everyone is covered. Covering everyone allows the allocation of resources based on the needs of a community instead of profitability. This kind of allocation of dollars allows for long range goals and planning to improve the health of a neighborhood, a community, a city, and a nation.

Portability means you can take it with you. U.S. citizens stay in unwanted jobs just to keep their health insurance. Canadians are free to follow their dreams. People are free to go where they want when they want, because coverage is guaranteed. Productivity of people who hate their jobs can stagnate an economy. This we should know better than any other nation.

Accessibility means freedom from barriers to health care. There are all kinds of barriers to care whether they are economic, geographic, or bureaucratic. They can all limit care with serious results. The Canada Health Act stipulates there must be accessibility, which means no barriers to care. How could Canada have gotten it so right?

In the United States, we have always maintained an arrogance about our ability to solve problems, to be the best at what we do. "Yankee ingenuity," don't you know. A problem is never solved until we put our spin on it. Perhaps this is why we chose to go off in our own direction when the rest of the world began to seek ways to provide health care for their populations. When at the end of World War II the United States and Canada both faced rising costs and needs for health care, Canada found a comprehensive solution. How they came to that solution and their current struggle to maintain it is the subject of this book. How that solution could solve the problems we face in the United States is the challenge before us. We have never turned away from a battle when the cause is just. Doesn't every U.S. citizen deserve decent health care? We cannot leave politics to just the politicians. It was the ordinary people who believed in a cause who shaped this nation. It will be the voting, the demanding, the protesting, the unrelenting U.S. public that will get health care for this nation. It will not be the politicians worried about campaign contributions and the next election. It will be angry citizens who become involved in the process, who write letters, make phone calls, and speak out at public forums who will make this change. The time is ripe for a change.

Claudia Fegan,
Chicago, November, 1997

I

A Canadian Love Affair

Ask any Canadian, "What is the difference between Canada and the United States?" Virtually every one of them will say "health care."

A remarkable 96 percent of Canadians prefer their health care system to the U.S. model.[1] And this support is not simply a reflection of Canadian nationalism in the face of a very large neighbor, although medicare certainly plays a central role as a "defining national characteristic."[2] Over the years, poll after poll has repeatedly demonstrated that health care is Canada's best-loved social program. An overwhelming majority of Canadians persistently say they want to keep their health care system.

In 1994, the Canadian government appointed a National Forum on Health to examine the current state and future possibilities of the health system. The focus groups and surveys conducted by the forum found that "the provision of health care services continues to receive strong and passionate support" among Canadians.[3] Similarly, the president of a major polling firm reported recently that among government programs "only the health care system received approval from a majority of Canadians." He went on to point out that the support even crosses social class lines. Otherwise strong differences in class values "don't occur to the same extent in the area of health care, perhaps because everyone can see themselves as becoming sick at some point."[4]

The current system is so popular that all Canadian politicians represent themselves as defenders of this sacred trust. Perhaps more surprisingly, so do many corporations in the private sector. Indeed, a major health insurance company has declared in a recent advertisement that it "believes strongly in the sanctity of Canadian medicare."[5]

The most important explanation for this support can be found in what are known as the five principles of the Canada Health Act. These are criteria for funding set out by the federal government, criteria the provinces* must follow in order to receive financial support for their health care services. Simply put, these principles require that core medical services be universal, portable, accessible, comprehensive, and publicly administered. In other words, all Canadians must have access to the medical services they require. These services must include all that is medically necessary, and must be provided regardless of age, prior condition, location, or employment. And they must be provided without regard to ability to pay. Canadian medicare was designed to allocate care on the basis of need, not individual finances.

And it worked. The system has delivered on the promised access to care. While "the number of uninsured Americans had risen to more than 40 million"[6] in 1995, virtually every Canadian is covered for essential care. This contrast in access to care can be traced to the basic philosophical approach used to fund services in Canada. As one 1981 task force put it, "Canadians are endeavouring to develop a health care system directed at health needs—not a competitive system to serve an illness market."[7]

This is made possible by the single-payer system. For the most part, health care in Canada is not *provided* by the government. It is *paid for* by governments. It is a public insurance system, a system in which governments at various levels pay for health services. Most of these services themselves are provided by nonprofit organizations or by doctors working on a fee-for-service basis. It is public payment for private practice and private provision.[8] This single-payer system has made care in Canada cheaper than in the United States, both because it signifi-

---

*Canada has a federal system with ten provinces and two (soon to be three) territories, each with its own health department. Although huge in size, the territories are tiny in population terms. Throughout this book "provinces" will be used to refer to both provinces and territories.

cantly reduces administrative costs and because it allows for more coherent management of services.

Until medicare was introduced, Canadian health care costs were growing as fast as those in the United States. But "the period of the most rapid escalation *ended* with the establishment of universal coverage"[9] paid for from public funds. Even more startling is the fact that *public* spending on health care accounts for virtually the same proportion of each country's total economy. Yet, Canada covers the whole population and the United States covers only the elderly, the very poor, the military, and some of the disabled.

With the government as the main purchaser of services, health care is not only cheaper for individual taxpayers. It is also cheaper for employers, especially for those employers facing unions strong enough to successfully demand full health care coverage. In the United States, Chrysler pays more for health care than it pays for steel.[10] In Canada, Chrysler does not have to pay for basic hospital or medical costs and therefore its employee costs are lower. Workers' compensation in Canada does not have to cover these basic costs either, and thus this protection too is cheaper for the Canadian employer.

With the single-payer scheme for many essential services, Canadians have a one-tier system. The rich and the poor go to the same hospitals and doctors. Neither receives a bill and the rich cannot buy quicker access, preferred status, or better facilities. What is covered by the public insurance system cannot be covered by a private insurer and doctors are not allowed to bill above the prescribed rate for services covered by the public insurance. Sharing facilities and services means that the entire population has a vested interest in maintaining the quality of care.

For more than a quarter century, Canada has been providing this comprehensive, accessible and high-quality care, without billing individuals for services or relating care to financial status. Equally important, it has done so more efficiently and at least as effectively as the competitive system serving an illness market in the United States. It is not surprising, then, that 96 per cent of Canadians prefer their system to the American way. It is somewhat more surprising that a majority of Americans also prefer the Canadian system to that in the United

3

States.[11] After all, health care services are very similar on both sides of the border.

In both countries, hospitals form the core of the system. And an operating room in one country looks much like one in the other. Hospitals in both countries offer high-tech services. On both sides of the border, most hospitals are owned by non-government organizations and function largely as independent entities. Hospitals in both countries vary in size and degree of specialization, although teaching hospitals across the continent tend to be large and diverse. Once in the door, it would be difficult to tell Toronto Hospital from the hospital in *Chicago Hope*.

Similarly, it would be difficult to identify which doctors are Canadian and which are American. Not only do both kinds wear white coats and stethoscopes, but the majority of doctors are paid on a fee-for-service basis. They are formally governed by agencies primarily made up of peers, intended to protect both patients and providers. Across North America, specialties are very similar and so are medical techniques. Indeed, research is freely shared and even jointly conducted across the border. Like hospitals, doctors' offices look virtually the same in Canada and the United States. Marcus Welby could be a Canadian.

Although doctors in both countries have fought hard to gain a monopoly over diagnosis and other medical practices, most of the actual patient care is provided by nurses of various kinds. Even the categories of nurses are basically the same on both sides of the border, as is their range of skills. Nurses are the main care providers both in and out of the hospital setting.

The settings where nurses and others provide care include long-term care facilities of various sorts. Homes for the elderly, nursing homes, and group homes are common everywhere in North America. And in both countries a great deal of care is provided in the home, often with assistance from home care nurses or other aides.

If health care is so similar in both countries, why is there such a strong preference for the Canadian system evident across the border as well as at home? Again, the explanation can be found mainly in the five principles on which Canadian health care delivery is based. And these in turn are related to the single-payer system and the insistence on one-tier delivery. They offer the most likely reasons for both Canadians and Americans preferring the Canadian approach. It is these principles, then, that are the subject matter of this book.

2
How Canadians Got Universal Coverage

In 1910, a six-year-old Scottish boy named Tommy Douglas got pneumonia. Then he fell and cut his knee on a stone. That cut changed Canadian history.

The small cut would not heal and Tommy developed a bone infection called osteomyelitis. Assisted by Tommy's mother and grandmother, the local doctor cleared the kitchen table and operated on his knee. The operation provided only temporary relief, however. After emigrating to Canada, Tommy found himself in a charity ward facing the amputation of the infected leg.

By chance, an orthopedic surgeon came across young Tommy. Seeing the opportunity for a useful teaching project, the surgeon sought permission to operate from Tommy's parents. The operation was such a success it surprised even the surgeon. Thanks to the surgeon's intervention Tommy went on to become something of an athlete, winning amateur boxing tournaments. In 1944, he also became the Premier of Saskatchewan, the province in western Canada that was to serve as the model for medicare.

According to his biographer, "The Medicare program of Saskatchewan when Tommy was Premier came directly from the fear of a poor boy that he would lose his leg, and a sense of the unfair caprice that saved it for him."[1] Audiences across the province, and across the country, heard Tommy Douglas explain that "When I thought about it, I realized that the same kind of service I got by a stroke of luck should have been available to every child in that ward, and not just to a case that looked like a good specimen for exhibition to medical students."

Tommy made the same kind of service available to every child and adult in his province. In the process, he demonstrated to Canadians that it was possible to base health care provision on shared responsibility and planning, rather than on luck.

A Tiny Province and a Tiny Man Lead the Way

Tommy Douglas started with the hospitals. The same year that Tommy cut his leg the Carnegie Foundation commissioned Abraham Flexner to tour Canada as well as the United States in order to assess medical schools. Flexner was not very pleased with what he found and offered a wide range of recommendations that were taken very seriously in both countries. In fact, the Flexner Report marked a turning point in medical education and in hospital practices. Science became firmly established as the basis for medicine and care became increasingly hospital-based.

By 1920, quality and standards in hospitals had improved significantly across North America. Many of the new technologies and treatments were too expensive for most individual doctors to purchase on their own, and it made more sense to deliver them within institutions where equipment and personnel could be shared. Hospitals became more and more popular. But they also became increasingly expensive. As a result, attention on both sides of the border shifted away from a primary concern with standards towards a concern with how to pay for hospital care.[2]

The Great Depression of the 1930s meant that many could not afford hospital care. It also meant that hospitals and care providers faced severe financial difficulties. In Canada and the United States, doctors and hospitals organized voluntary insurance programs to help cover patient hospital expenses. In both countries, Blue Cross emerged during this period as a major institution for insuring hospital care. Nevertheless, high unemployment and low wages meant that many still remained without coverage for hospital services. This was particularly the case for the elderly and the disabled.[3]

With the Second World War came a growing demand for hospital care and significant advances in the kinds of medical treatment that could best be delivered in those hospitals. While governments were committed to providing care for their returning wounded, many more required the kind of care they could not afford but could see available to others. In the aftermath of depression and war, there was in Canada and elsewhere "a mood of rebellion against the universal risks of unemployment and sickness, disability and old age, widowhood and poverty," combined with an unwillingness to see these risks as the fault or responsibility of individuals.[4] Together, these developments set the stage for government intervention in health care. And they set the stage for Tommy Douglas's party in Saskatchewan.

Two and a half years after its 1944 election victory, Tommy Douglas's government introduced North America's first universal hospital insurance scheme. And the Saskatchewan Government did this in a poor province that was heavily in debt and had a rapidly growing hospital admission rate as well as a severe shortage of hospital beds, doctors, and nurses. Moreover, the Government had no model to follow for such a scheme and had only limited data on actual costs.

Hospital Insurance for All in Saskatchewan

Nevertheless, a universal hospital insurance scheme came into effect on January 1, 1947. Everyone in the province was covered for inpatient care, regardless of financial resources or location. There was no limitation on the number of days a patient could stay in the hospital, as long as the stay was medically necessary.

No bill was paid at the door or arrived in the mail after a patient went home. The only payment was a per capita tax or premium that offered no choice about opting out. Initially set at $5.00 a year, the premium was very low. It could however mean a heavy burden for large households. To address this problem, the Government set an annual cap of $30.00 per family. Some categories of people, such as those who had already been covered by virtue of military service, disability, poverty, or old age, were not required to pay the premium, and no resident of the province was refused care.

Hospital costs were paid by the government, based on a formula that took both the size of the institution and the number of its patients into account. The premiums paid by residents were supplemented by general tax revenues. This was designed to ensure that all hospitals were paid for their operating expenses. The guarantee of government support also meant that people could count on their hospital, without fear that it would close due to financial difficulties.

The experiment worked. The success of the plan was demonstrated in the 1948 election that returned Tommy Douglas and his party to power. It was the most widely accepted government program and few people openly objected to paying their premiums. The number of hospital beds grew rapidly and so did their utilization.

Of course there was opposition from those who reject government intervention in any form and from those who disagreed with Tommy's view that health services are "an inalienable right of being a citizen."[5] There was also concern about the high rate of utilization. This use, however, was primarily explained by the backlog that had built up under previous shortages, by transportation difficulties that limited the use of house calls and by the lack of alternative institutional care.[6] The plan did cost more than was estimated but this may have primarily reflected the inadequacies of the data on which the estimates were based. As we shall see, in the long run public hospital insurance provided cheaper care than private plans, and did so without creating individual financial hardship. Equally important, hospitals accepted everyone and allowed them to stay as long as they needed care.

The Model Catches On

Politicians, bureaucrats, and academics from across the country and around the world flocked to see the Saskatchewan plan in action. Like Saskatchewan, other jurisdictions had become involved in health care in various ways over the years because individual finances and private insurance plans were inadequate. And like Saskatchewan, they were faced with populations that expected, and demanded, a better life after the sacrifices of war. This was particularly the case in relation to health care.

Several provinces had introduced some form of hospital insurance around the same time as Saskatchewan, with varying degrees of success. Although hospital cost and utilization rates were rising in these provinces, they were not rising faster than costs in provinces without any government plans. Indeed, there was evidence that government plans were already controlling costs, a trend that interested the provinces without health care plans.

In Canada's most western province, British Columbia, costs under the universal government plan grew more slowly than in Ontario.[7] Yet Ontario was a large, industrialized province enjoying significant economic growth, albeit without a public hospital insurance scheme. In Ontario, the situation in terms of coverage was similar to the current one in the United States. Some people were covered as individuals through their union contracts and other employee plans. Some were covered through individual or cooperatively organized insurance schemes. Some had no coverage at all, unless they were indigent and the government offered care through a welfare program.

Research in Ontario demonstrated that there were significant limits to the number of people who could be covered by voluntary employee plans. Such plans mainly worked when people had secure employment and when premiums were deducted automatically from the payroll. Even then, people were not assured full coverage when they entered hospital. The larger the bill, the smaller the proportion covered by the plan. This was particularly the case if coverage was provided by a for-profit firm.[8] When insurance did not provide coverage, governments were increasingly expected to assume the burden.

Provincial governments were not only concerned about individual coverage and their costs. They were also concerned about hospital deficits, deficits that provincial governments were pressured to cover. A 1954 report found that voluntary insurance plans were part of the problem rather than part of the solution. According to the *Taylor Report*, insurance schemes added significantly to hospital expenditures: "eighteen percent in the case of Blue Cross, thirty percent in commercial group contracts, seventy percent in commercial individual contracts, and sixteen percent in the case of cooperatives."[9] Moreover, although the insured went more often to hospitals than the uninsured, the uninsured stayed much longer. The uninsured often cost more as a result. Their costs were borne by the provinces because no one else was willing or able to pick up the tab. Clearly, more individual insurance schemes were not the answer to controlling provincial costs, especially not schemes of the commercial variety.

But provinces were having difficulty paying for hospital costs. While health care was a provincial responsibility, the federal government had the financial resources. The main taxing power rested at the national level. Moreover, provinces varied enormously both in their ability to raise money and in their demands for health services. In largely rural provinces, for example, hospital coverage was more difficult to provide than was the case in highly urban centers. It was not surprising then that the provinces turned to the federal government for support in providing hospital care.

Developing a National Hospital Insurance Plan

The federal government had tried to initiate a national program right after the Second World War but the project was abandoned when the provinces could not reach agreement. In the meantime, however, the federal government supported research on illness that clearly established both the link between low income and poor health and the disproportionate financial burden placed on those who were ill. In spite of their better health, the higher income groups received more care. The same kinds of pattern were evident among rich and poor provinces. There was significant inequality among provinces in terms of facilities, services, and access.

Even though the provinces had responsibility for health care, national health strategy did not begin and end with research. The federal government also offered money to support capital expenditures on hospitals. Ten years after the war, then, there were many more hospitals but there was no more money to operate them. What the provinces did have were rising costs, research demonstrating that privately organized insurance schemes were inadequate, and the example of Saskatchewan.

11

They went for the Saskatchewan model. In sharp contrast to recent U.S. proposals, the federal–provincial plan was really very simple, consisting of a six-page federal act. It laid out a clear way forward. Once a majority of the provinces representing a majority of the population agreed, the federal government would pay approximately half of the cost of normal maintenance and operating expenditures for hospital care and for services in aid of diagnosis in hospitals. Just how the provinces delivered care was left up to them.

To qualify for this financial support, provinces were required to make this care universally available to all their residents. Everyone must be able to get in, and out, without having to pay to sign up or to move. The Prime Minister of the day made it clear that universally available meant "all citizens of that province are able to take advantage of the contribution we are to make from general tax revenue." Moreover, this availability "must be real, not just theoretical." Equally important, it "must not only be available to all but generally utilized."[10]

In other words, hospital care must be not only universal but also accessible. And to be accessible it had to be comprehensive and provided under the same conditions for everyone. These requirements are discussed in greater detail in later chapters. It is important to note here, however, that the planners recognized the critical links among these three principles. They are not factors to be traded off, played against each other or implemented one by one. There was little point in establishing a universal plan if it contained obstacles preventing some residents from using its services or if it contained only some of the services they would need. A universal, accessible, and comprehensive plan makes the full range of required services readily available to all.

April 1957 marked a truly momentous development in Canadian history. Unbelievable as it may seem in this huge and often divided country, all three federal political parties unanimously supported legislation establishing a national hospital-insurance program. Both the House of Commons and the Senate unanimously voted for the legislation. This rare unanimity did not mean there had been no opponents to the program. Indeed, Canadian hospital insurance had many of the same kinds of adversaries that are vocal in the United States today. But the unanimity did reflect the strong popular support for the initiative and the compromises that had eventually led to its introduction.

Not all hospitals were in favor of the plan. As is the case in the United States, few hospitals were government owned and many of those operating the hospitals feared a government takeover by means of a public insurance plan. Their fears were largely addressed by a program that left these hospitals virtually unchanged in structure and ownership. Governments merely promised to pay for the care the hospitals provided. Thus these hospitals had a guarantee of payment, placing them on solid financial ground while allowing them to practice in much the same way as they had before public insurance. For the most part, the governing structures of the hospitals were left in place. The Hospital Insurance and Diagnostic Services Act did require that they meet certain standards, but most had been doing so already. The difference was in the billing. Now they had only one payer for most expenditures and a lot less paperwork.

Others had feared that patients would rush to the hospitals once service was free. But no such rush occurred. Instead, the annual rate of increase initially declined. Compared to the hospitals in the United States, the decline was even greater.[11] The sharp increase in hospital use in both Canada and the United States had begun *before* public insurance, when hospitals became better at providing care and significantly improved their reputations. In Canada, the effect of public hospital insurance was to moderate use while guaranteeing universal coverage. This response should not be surprising. Few people really want to get into a hospital simply because it is free. When there is no profit to be gained for hospitals by filling up wards with patients who do not need care and when funding is stabilized, there is also less incentive for hospitals to actively seek patients.

It is important to note, though, that the government ignored advice from the Canadian Hospital Association that might have further reduced hospital use in the long run. This Association suggested that introducing hospital insurance alone would encourage people to use hospitals rather than other, more appropriate services. The organization therefore suggested that the plan include additional types of care, such as nursing homes, home care, homes for the aged, and convales-

13

cent homes. The government failed to take this advice, a decision that led to cost increases over time and a growing emphasis on hospital-based care.

The medical profession also opposed the introduction of public hospital insurance. This was a reversal of its earlier position taken during more difficult financial times. While the doctors were happy to have the government pick up the tab for those who could not pay for insurance, they did not want the government to control all hospital insurance. By the 1950s the doctors were having less difficulty getting their patients into hospitals and doctors themselves had been active in establishing voluntary hospital insurance plans.

The government did not accept the position of organized medicine on universal hospital insurance but did leave the doctors in charge of hospital admissions and use. The government also left their fee-for-services practices untouched. For most medical practitioners, the public insurance plan simply meant in the end that they did not have to consider the patient's income when ordering hospital care. Instead, they could base their decisions on medical need. And they could do so with considerably less paperwork than they had in the past with multiple plans.

Other health providers had been more supportive of public hospital insurance. Rarely in a position to bill patients directly, these mainly female providers had much to gain from stable, and public, financing. With secure funding and more secure employment, these women were in a position to demand better wages and conditions of work. The numbers of jobs for women in hospital grew dramatically. Throughout the 1960s, unions emerged in the hospital sector and managed to significantly improve the employment conditions of hospital workers. In the case of registered nurses in Quebec, for example, wages ranged from $10 to $20 for a 54-hour week in 1946, and the nurses had no paid vacation, maternity leave, or pension. By 1966, they had salaries ranging from $85 to $109 for a 36.25-hour week and they were eligible for four weeks' paid vacation, maternity leave, and pensions.[12]

Commercial insurance companies were less thrilled about the public plan. As was the case in the United States, nonprofit plans had been popular but the for-profit share of the market was growing rapidly

14

during the 1950s . Health care was increasingly seen as a money maker, a place to make huge profits. Yet many were without coverage while others made great sacrifices to pay premiums that too often left them without necessary care. The association representing insurance officers suggested that they could address the problem of undue hardship for low-income people by introducing a premium scheme graduated by income. The association also suggested that the government support voluntary insurance by following the American model of allowing individuals to deduct premiums from their taxes.

This tax deduction approach is simply another way of providing government financing, only in this method the government has less say about how the money is spent and who gets care. The government would forgo taxes but would retain all the problems of uneven and inadequate benefits in place. At the same time, tax deductions would provide even more government support for wealthier citizens while offering no help to those with incomes too low to benefit from tax deduction schemes.

With research and experience demonstrating the weaknesses in the association's approach, the federal government rejected these proposals from the insurance companies. Under the legislation it introduced, the insurance companies were not allowed to cover the hospital care already covered under the public plan. They could not compete with the public insurance scheme. But the government did try to placate them in another way. The private insurance companies could still cover the extras. These included slightly different things in different provinces, but in all provinces included at least some dental work, some prescription drugs taken outside the hospital setting, and some supplementary coverage for care provided outside Canada. In all provinces, then, there remained plenty of room for continued insurance sales.

No province could resist the federal offer of cash to help pay for hospital insurance, or the demands from citizens and the evidence of the research. By 1961 all provinces had hospital insurance in place and almost all Canadians were covered by a public plan. The precise nature of the plans varied from province to province because the provincial governments remained the chief decision-makers in health care. At the same time, the very substantial differences in hospital services that had preceded federal intervention were largely eliminated. Hospital services became more equal across Canada and among individuals. Canadian residents could walk into a hospital, present their hospital card or health number, and be admitted. They neither saw the bill nor paid directly for the basic services, no matter how often or how long they used them. Tommy Douglas's dream of free hospital care came true. To this day, Canadians overwhelmingly share his view that the tax system is the most equitable, as well as the most efficient, way to pay for hospital services.

Medical Insurance

Tommy's dream did not stop with hospitals, however. The surgeon who had taken him on as a charity case would still not have been covered by the public hospital insurance plan. Tommy would still have been at risk. Determined to make care truly universal, Tommy took on medicine next. And this proved to be a much bigger battle.

Doctors were not nearly as keen on or complaisant about public medical insurance as they had been about hospital insurance. Like those in the United States, Canadian doctors in the 1950s and 1960s worked primarily as independent professionals. Medical decisions were assumed to be based exclusively on the scientific knowledge of the doctors, without regard for financial or other constraints. Doctors did piecework, charging patients for each individual treatment, diagnosis, and visit. In theory, they could charge or order whatever they wanted. In practice, they were constrained not only by the limited financial resources of many of their patients but also by insurance company regulations.

In theory, doctors' incomes were unlimited. In practice, however, patients often could not or would not pay and insurance companies often had fee schedules and maximums on payouts. Billing was an enormous expense and bad debts were common. As a result of the fee-for-service system, doctors' incomes varied enormously, in terms of what any individual might earn in a given year and in terms of what different doctors earned. Few doctors had guaranteed jobs or payments.

16

Not all doctors did piecework or practiced alone. In both countries, some doctors were employed in group practices or in community clinics where salaries were the norm. As well, some were hired by hospitals or municipalities on a salaried basis. On occasion, doctors were forced to take salaries because they could not survive on the earnings from their independent practices. This was particularly the case in rural areas with sparse populations and low incomes, as well as in those urban areas with high concentrations of people living on low incomes. There were certainly doctors who preferred the stability of a salary, and the possibility it offered for a focus on prevention rather than cure. But most doctors were strongly committed to the fee-for-service payment scheme and to solo practice. Public health care insurance was a red flag to many of these bulls.

At first glance, Saskatchewan doctors seemed different. A much higher proportion of them worked in clinics and on salary. The town of Swift Current, for example, had a clinic very much like the Kaiser plans in California and the New York Health Insurance Plan. Like them, it offered high-quality care paid for on a per capita basis in a manner that gave both patients and doctors considerable choice. Indeed, throughout Saskatchewan there was a tradition of engaging in clinics "municipal doctors" who were paid on a combination of salary and fee-for-service. Their experience with this system had led many doctors to support an approach based on salaried, group work in clinics. In addition, Saskatchewan doctors had repeatedly endorsed a public health insurance scheme throughout the 1940s and had been active in the development of the hospital insurance scheme. The successful pioneering by the province of public hospital insurance had both reflected and reinforced the strong cooperative tradition in Saskatchewan. Conditions seemed ripe for a medical insurance scheme, and quite different from those in most of Canada or in the United States.

But it did not work out that way. Although doctors had suffered financially during the Great Depression and immediately after the war, in the 1950s Saskatchewan doctors enjoyed among the highest incomes in the country. Doctors had become very active in voluntary plans, even organizing coverage themselves. Such plans were increasingly seen by them as the better way. By the time medical insurance pro-

17

posals were seriously put on the table, many doctors wanted the government to stick to covering the old and the poor, leaving the rest to them. They shared with many doctors across North America the fear that government intervention would mean loss of control over clinical decisions. Equating fee-for-service with independence, they saw any universal public plan as state medicine that would place them under bureaucratic control and reduce their incomes. This was particularly the case for the significant number of doctors who came to Saskatchewan in order to avoid Britain's National Health Service. Public insurance could also mean more demands for public involvement in health care planning, in areas where doctors had dominated the scene. Many feared a public plan would undermine their power.

So when the Saskatchewan government campaigned on a medical insurance program, the doctors launched their own counter-campaign. Like doctors in the United States, those in Canada had become accustomed to power and to having their say. They had also become well organized through their colleges and medical associations. Although they could not always count on public support, they did know that patients need their services and become very nervous when these services are denied. Recognizing this, Tommy Douglas made many concessions to the doctors in developing his policy.

He remained firmly committed, however, to public, universal insurance. Any young Tommy would now receive care without question. When he designed the legislation establishing the first universal medical insurance scheme in 1961, Tommy made sure the scheme was public and compulsory, in spite of the doctors' strong resistance. Every resident had to belong and every resident had the right to necessary medical care. This care included the services of physicians and surgeons, whether these services were provided in the hospital, the office, or the home. As was the case with hospital insurance, small premiums were paid, with a maximum per family, but most of the money came from general tax revenue.

Like hospital insurance, it was a payment scheme rather than a delivery scheme. None of the dire things doctors predicted came true. Doctors could continue to practice the way they had in the past, except now the bills would be automatically paid by the government and no doctor was unemployed or underemployed. Under the public insurance scheme, and contrary to the doctors' claims, their clinical decisions were not questioned or even monitored. The College of Physicians and Surgeons controlled by the doctors was still completely in charge of ethical concerns. In the face of doctor resistance, Tommy had given up on the idea of making group practice the central feature of the scheme. Doctors could continue to practice alone and to practice anywhere in the province they wished.

The doctors won on fee-for-service, too. In their view, this protected the independence of their clinical decisions. Moreover, payment from the government did not mean that the government determined who the patients were. Doctors could reject patients without penalty or surveillance from government bureaucrats. Patients, too, were able to choose. They could move freely from doctor to doctor. The main effect of the introduction of medical insurance was that neither doctors nor patients had to make finances a primary concern.

In spite of these concessions, the majority of doctors rejected the Saskatchewan legislation. And they went much farther than the usual practices of lobbying and writing editorial complaints. Unthinkable as it had seemed for this profession, the doctors went on strike and many threatened to leave the province for good. The battle was very bitter and very long. The doctors and their political allies used every kind of tactic imaginable, building on the insecurities people feel when health care is absent. Mothers were told their children were threatened, women were told their health records would become public documents, and the population in general was told medicare was a communist plot.[13] The strike brought further minor concessions from the Government but no overall victory for the doctors' demands, demands that were primarily about keeping the old system and doctors' power in place. A universal system, supported by taxes and administered by a public body, had come to Saskatchewan.

Ironically perhaps, doctors were among those who benefited the most. Their incomes increased by 35 percent in 1963, making them the highest-paid physicians in Canada and the only ones with a public medical insurance scheme.[14] They had guaranteed payment, guaranteed employment and lots of choice. They had significantly less paperwork and seldom had to spend time discussing finances with patients. Of course, the doctors were not the only opponents of a public plan. The for-profit insurance companies also sought to defend the growing market in health care coverage. Their interests did not precisely coincide with those of the doctors, however, given that the doctors wanted more independence from surveillance of any sort. The insurance companies had little support from the voters, either. The public plan was intended to eliminate insurance practices such as deductibles and limitations related to age, employment, or membership in particular groups. Why would voters prefer a system that had higher premiums, offered less coverage, and discriminated on the basis of a wide variety of conditions beyond individual control, rather than one which promised to cover everyone, regardless of history, condition, or ability to pay? It became clear in Saskatchewan that the voters were prepared to pay somewhat higher taxes in order to have a universal, public plan.

Universal Medical Care

Once again, Saskatchewan had led the way. It had demonstrated that universal medical coverage was not just a dream but a real possibility in practice. Even the doctors, through their Canadian Medical Association (CMA), had to admit that the majority of the population seemed to support a plan that covered medical services through taxation.

It was this same medical association that had successfully pressured the federal government to establish a Royal Commission on Health Services. Such commissions are a Canadian tradition, and often serve as much to divert attention from an issue as they do to solve contentious problems or take new initiatives. It was not surprising, then, that it was a Conservative government that responded to the CMA request. It was more surprising when the Royal Commission rejected the doctors' preference for voluntary plans supplemented by government subsidies for the poor. Instead, the Royal Commission called for a universal medical scheme based on Tommy Douglas's initial proposals and for immediate action to get it implemented across Canada.

There were two major reasons for the Royal Commission's recommendations. First, Saskatchewan had proven it could be done. Second, the research clearly demonstrated that a public plan was not only the most popular route but also the most efficient and effective, especially if equity were a concern. The Royal Commission concluded that a voluntary plan would take too long to develop and would necessarily be incomplete, leaving too many people without coverage. A subsidy plan would require applying means tests regularly to huge sectors of the population, incurring enormous administrative costs as well as very large subsidy costs. For adequate care, the majority of the population would end up being eligible for some kind of subsidy anyway. By subsidizing programs rather than people, governments could more cheaply cover the entire population. In addition, a single plan would make it easier to integrate services in ways that would not only be cost-effective but also more care-effective.

The Royal Commission was also convinced that a government plan need not reduce choice or limit democracy. Indeed, it could enhance democracy and choice by ensuring both universal rights to care and public decision-making. While the program would be compulsory, as long as the decisions were made by democratically elected legislatures public participation would be assured. Provinces could retain their right to organize health care in ways that responded to their particular needs and traditions. At the same time, equalization payments among provinces would ensure that provincial disparities in services and facilities were addressed. This, too, could enhance democratic choice by equalizing access across the land. Individuals would retain their right to choose their physician, only now the choice would not have to be based on ability to pay. Similarly, physicians would retain their right to locate where they wished. They could also accept or reject patients without regard to ability to pay.

In opting for a government insurance plan, the Royal Commission was in direct opposition to the insurance companies and the doctors represented by the CMA. In the face of the Saskatchewan initiative, these companies had launched a campaign against government insurance that began with getting the doctors on their side. They did so by pandering to the doctors' fear of government control and socialized medicine. While claiming commitment to health services for all, the insurance companies raised the spectre of a government monopoly that

21

would make doctors "prisoners" of bureaucracy, allowing govern-ments to "control the purse strings and dictate the terms of service."[15]

In the view of the insurance industry, the only democratic alterna-tive was multiple insurance companies offering voluntary plans. In other words, they wanted an open market for themselves. Not surpris-ingly, the insurance companies failed to address either the monopoly tendencies in their industry or industry efforts to limit expenditures through bureaucratic restrictions and controls over doctors. Yet in the United States, insurance companies have become large oligopolies, controlling the market for insurance both in terms of areas of the coun-try and in terms of services offered. Individuals have less and less choice about the companies or the services. Doctors too have less and less choice about what services to provide, as insurance and other managed care companies increasingly dictate the terms under which care can be provided through control of the purse strings. According to one re-searcher, "All forms of managed care represent attempts to control costs by modifying the behavior of doctors."[16]

From the Royal Commission's perspective, democracy and the in-surance companies' notion of choice could be accommodated by cov-ering basic services solely under the compulsory government plan. Insurance for additional services beyond the basics could be offered by any insurance company. Individuals would have free choice in cover-ing extras beyond the standard services. They could for example, buy coverage for more physiotherapy or home care than that provided as part of the standard care package.

The Royal Commission also dealt directly with the industry's appeal to doctors. Instead of fees determined by insurance companies, the Royal Commission offered fees established through negotiations be-tween the doctors' associations and governments. Although doctors claimed to have choice about fee schedules, in practice fees had been set by insurance companies and by colleges of physicians and surgeons. So the proposal for a public insurance scheme based on fee-for-service did not constitute that much of a departure from past practices and retained more power for the doctors than may have been the case under private insurance plans. Indeed, with all doctors negotiating col-lectively with one body, they had much more power than when individually negotiating with insurance companies or even individual patients.

Doctors could not, however, easily see the threat from insurance companies. Many remained fundamentally opposed to government compulsory plans, in spite of the evidence indicating that a public, single-payer scheme could bring them, and the patients they served, significant medical, administrative, and economic benefits. Like many doctors in the United States today, they stood firmly committed to what they saw as a free market in care. The efforts by doctors and insurance companies to prevent a public insurance scheme for medical services were not without initial success. Unlike later surveys taken after Canadians had some experience with their medicare scheme, a 1965 poll found only a minority of the country's residents in favor of a compulsory plan.[17]

In contrast to the insurance companies and the doctors, the labor movement strongly endorsed a universal medical plan. Health care, in the view of labor, was a public service rather than a market one. Labor agreed with the Royal Commission that government coverage of basic services was the only way to ensure democratic choice in ways that would put citizens' interests before those of the insurance companies. Fiddling with the current system was rejected not only on the grounds of commitment to social responsibility but also on the grounds of efficiency. In labor's view, insurance schemes based on principles such as deductibles and other financial contributions were both antithetical to democracy and administratively expensive.

At an earlier period in U.S. history, some unions had opposed a public plan on the grounds that it would undermine the benefits workers gained from belonging to a union that won health care coverage for its members. However, the Depression had made it clear in both countries that labor alone could not protect citizens from disastrous health costs. Moreover, "With the official recognition of organized labour's right to represent workers, one of the reasons for opposing social insurance disappeared."[18] The Canadian labor movement fought hard for a public system. Like the insurance companies, however, it was not left out of the picture by the new system. Under the recommendations

23

of the Royal Commission, unions could still bargain for the extras as part of their collective agreements.

While the employers of these union members did not campaign for a public system, with the exception of the insurance companies they did not vigorously campaign against one either. Large employers facing strong unions were increasingly signing collective agreements that made medical care a bargained right. This benefit was expensive. As we have seen, in the United States, Chrysler and the other auto makers pay more for health care benefits for their current and former employees than they do for steel. In Canada, the public system shared the costs among all taxpayers and, in the process made care cheaper for everyone, including employers. Indeed, according to the World Economic Forum, public health care is a major factor in making Canadian employers competitive.[19] Chrysler, for example, calculated that in 1988 health benefits cost it $US 700 a car in the United States and $US 233 a car in Canada.[20] Meanwhile in the United States, according to one estimate, "the major issue in three strike actions out of four from 1989 to 1992 was health care benefits."[21] Thus it is not surprising that large Canadian employers were not united in strong opposition against a public insurance plan.

In spite of the compromises it made and the model of Saskatchewan's success, the federal government had more trouble with insurance for doctors than it had had with insurance for hospitals. A vocal and organized opposition meant the vote in the federal parliament was not unanimous. Mainly because many provinces seemed reluctant, this time there was no requirement that a majority sign up for the plan before it came into effect. But once again the promise of money worked. The offer to pay half of costs for insured medical services was an offer the provinces could not long resist.

As was the case with hospital insurance, the plan was quite simple. The Medical Care Act of 1966 covered eight pages. And as with hospital insurance, the legislation required only that provinces meet some basic principles in order to get the money. In plain language, the Act said all citizens must have access to necessary medical care, without regard to income or any other conditions. These principles were very much like those for hospital insurance.

Although it took a little longer than hospital insurance to spread from sea to sea, medical insurance was introduced in every province within five years. By the beginning of the 1970s, every Canadian was covered by both hospital and medical insurance. All Canadians had an insurance number or a health care card that gave them the right to services in the hospital or in the doctor's office.

In the beginning, it was simply an insurance plan that covered everyone. It was insurance with a difference, however. Not only was everyone covered, whatever their diagnosis or previous health, but there were no differences in costs to individuals. Three of the ten provinces required those who could to pay regular premiums, although in no case were these premiums connected to the services rendered.[22] The premiums did not vary according to age, health, or use of services. Everyone who paid a premium paid the same low rate, with special rates for families. The premiums were token contributions, however. They were more an ideological legacy from the past than a means of raising necessary revenue. Most of the money for medical care came out of general tax revenues and most of the patients never saw a bill.

As provinces became more experienced with their plans and less tied to old habits of insurance, they became increasingly aware of how silly it was to spend money collecting premiums and sorting out who should pay. Ontario, the province with the largest population, moved away from collecting premiums from individuals, leaving only Alberta and British Columbia collecting small portions of their health financing requirements in this way.

The notion of universal coverage included doctors, too. General practitioners (GPs) and specialists alike were covered under the plan. Whatever their location, doctors also remained fully in charge of their private practices, retaining virtually all the power they enjoyed under the old system. In fact, their power increased because many of them had more influence over government policy than they had had over private insurance schemes. Fees were negotiated by the provincial medical associations representing the doctors and were set at a level that ensured substantial incomes for them all. Because fees varied by service and speciality, specialists continued to earn significantly more than GPs. Thus, earning differentials similar to those existing before public insurance were retained.

Table 2.1
MEDICARE IN CANADA AND THE UNITED STATES 1996

	United States	Canada
Population Covered	people over 65	everyone
Hospital Insurance		
deductibles	$760 per benefit period	none
co-insurance	$190 per day for 61st to 90th day per benefit period from 91st to 150th day $380 per day but coverage beyond 90 days in any benefit period is limited to the number of lifetime reserve days available	none
skilled nursing facility co-insurance	$95 per day for 21st to 100th day per benefit period	none
hospital insurance premium	paid by those not eligible for social security $311 per month	none in 10 out of 12 jurisdictions★
Medical Insurance		
deductible	$100 per year	none
monthly premium	$43.80	none in 10 out of 12 jurisdictions★

★ Only the provinces of Alberta and British Columbia charged premiums. These premiums were quite low. For example, in 1997 Alberta charged $34 a month to individuals and $68 a month to families for combined hospital and medical coverage, with subsidies for those with very low incomes.

Source: "Medicare Deductible, Coinsurance and Premium Amounts," *The Federal Register,* 61:214 (November 1996), pp. 55002–009.

In spite of these benefits, many doctors still feared a public scheme. Strike action and promises to leave Canada were once again on the agenda. Although such threats were not more powerful than the federal money offer, many provinces did make further concessions in an attempt to placate the medical profession. Still militant, some doctors carried out their threat to leave the country. Other doctors followed less public and visible forms of resistance. Under the terms initially set out by most provinces, the doctors had the right to opt out of the plan and bill patients directly. A significant number did so at the beginning, preferring their private practice without direct public payment.

In most provinces, patients visiting these doctors were allowed to then bill the government in much the same way they had billed insurance companies. This doctor resistance to public insurance did not last for long, either. Like the provinces in the case of premiums, most doctors soon realized it was both simpler and cheaper to send all their bills directly to the government. The public plan reduced doctors' administrative costs because they had only one payer to bill. But medicare did more than reduce billing expenses. Given that doctors were guaranteed payment for all services rendered, it was not surprising that research in Quebec found that doctors' income went up after public medical insurance was introduced. Perhaps more surprising was the finding that their hours of work decreased as did the time they spent in house calls. Public payment clearly allowed doctors to manage their time, and finances, better.[23]

These conditions, along with the increasing government support for medical education, contributed to the increase in the number of doctors. It more than countered the small exodus that had followed immediately in the wake of public medical insurance. Between 1968 and 1983, Canada's overall population/physician ratio dropped from 909 to 603, and fully 35 percent of the increase consisted of doctors graduating from foreign medical schools.[24] Universal coverage nonetheless meant that doctors had more patients. More doctors helped ensure that patients had universal coverage at the same time as the government ensured that all doctors were paid. With medical insurance allowing patients to choose both when they saw a doctor and which doctors they saw, it was critical to provide an adequate supply of doctors to offer the services.

Although a majority of the doctors accepted the fees paid by government, a small group stuck to sending out bills. Some remained dissatisfied with the negotiated fee settlement, even though it meant more money and improved conditions. By the late 1970s, a growing number were "extra billing" for their services. They would, for example, charge to keep patient records or for house calls. Some would even demand that their patients pay an extra fee, above what the negotiated fee schedule provided for an insured service. These additional charges had to be paid by the individual, rather than by the government through the insurance plan. Extra billing threatened the very basis of the public plan. Tommy Douglas and the growing number of Canadians who had come to love the health care system, were alarmed. The basis of the plan was access without financial barriers. Extra billing clearly constituted a financial barrier.

The Canada Health Act

This time the battle was taken up by a woman. Quiet and "mortally shy," her friends at Teacher's College predicted she would marry an ambassador.[25] Instead, she was elected to Parliament and in 1977 was appointed by Prime Minister Pierre Trudeau as Minister of National Health and Welfare. In charge of the government department with the largest budget, Monique Bégin took on the doctors and the provinces. She won, and so did the people of Canada.

The stage for the battle was set by a new funding policy for health care. Like governments around the world, Canada had become concerned about rapidly rising health care costs. The commitment to pay half what provinces spent on specified services left the federal government without the means to plan overall expenses. The promise was open-ended from the federal perspective.

Although this plan kept costs below those in the United States, the federal government searched for ways to develop a more closed-ended approach to funding. It wanted to know what it would spend each year. The result, after lengthy negotiations with the provinces, was a new formula for payment and new choices for the provinces. Under the Established Programs Financing (EPF) Act, the federal government would transfer a lump sum to the provinces each year instead of paying half the bills. This cash transfer was supplemented by a transfer of tax points, that is, by giving the provinces the right to tax revenues that had previously been the exclusive property of the federal government. The agreement ensured continuing, and significant, federal financial support for health care, with less scrutiny from Ottawa.

No longer paying half the bills, the federal government no longer required the provinces to submit those bills before payment was made. The provinces thus had greater leeway in their spending and billing. So did the doctors.

Spectacular increases in incomes, guaranteed payments, and secure employment were still not enough for some doctors. Many were not satisfied with the quite generous fees negotiated with the provinces. With the more relaxed payment conditions now in place, a growing number began billing for extras. Some of the provincial governments and hospitals followed this example by charging patients small fees for publicly insured services.

Often defined by the doctors as part of their fight against socialism,[26] the additional billing was defined by others as a threat to medicare. The fundamental principle was that there should be no financial barrier to health care, and fees were a financial barrier.

Monique Bégin certainly defined the extra fees, which were imposed on individual patients when they received services, as constituting a financial barrier. The tall, elegant woman with a charming French accent when she speaks English has a wonderful sense of humor. She needed the charm, the humor, and an iron commitment to the fundamental principles of Canadian health care to take on such powerful opponents. She had all these qualities in abundance. Her goal was simple. Consolidate, and guarantee, what existed. Clearly, provinces and doctors were not voluntarily protecting the universal plan. Some sanctions were necessary. Given that the provinces had undertaken medicare in return for economic rewards, financial penalties seemed appropriate.

There was no question the public supported the plan in place. Poll after poll confirmed its popularity. Even letters from doctors indicated support for an enforcement strategy to keep the plan, albeit with one doctor in favor for every two against the proposal to impose financial sanctions on provinces allowing extra billing. Some of her opponents, though, were quite extreme. One doctor wrote to prescribe "hormones to combat my menopause, as it is clear you are crazy," she was later to recall.[27]

All the old tactics were dredged up and all the old players reemerged to battle over the new legislation. A media campaign developed, with many of the major newspapers opposing the proposal to impose sanctions. A doctors' strike was once more on the agenda. Once again, compromises were made to little effect in terms of the opposition. And yet another investigation done for the Government confirmed that the most efficient and effective means of ensuring universal care was a plan that did not require the collection of individual fees.[28]

In spite of the resistance, the federal minister and her colleagues in the Liberal Government held firm on the principle that there should be no financial barriers to health care. They went ahead and introduced the Canada Health Act to Parliament, where it was passed with unanimous consent in 1984. This legislation, which clearly enjoyed broad popular support, brought together hospital and medical insurance into a single, simple act. It clearly stated the commitment to the five principles provided in the earlier legislation: those of public administration, comprehensiveness, universality, portability and accessibility.

The Canada Health Act was somewhat longer than the two earlier pieces of legislation, although it still covered only thirteen pages. It was longer primarily because it set out definitions of the five principles and because it provided specific penalties for those provinces allowing extra fees. Basically, the Act stated that for every dollar citizens paid in user fees or extra billing, the federal government would deduct a dollar from its cash transfer to the province concerned. Everyone must be covered for medically necessary hospital and doctor services—no extra fees could be attached to these services.

The penalties worked. Provinces balked at first, as did the doctors, but eventually fees were forbidden in provincial jurisdictions. Canada finally had universal coverage for care, without regard to ability to pay and without individual patients having to pay fees for services.

The Canada Health Act was intended to do more than clarify the five principles, however. And it was designed to do more than prevent extra fees. It was also intended to help shift the focus away from curative procedures towards preventative strategies. As was the case in the

United States and in the rest of the Western world, health policy analysts in Canada were increasingly critical of care that was exclusively hospital-and doctor-centered. Part of the idea was to encourage a broader range of services and approaches in the public system. Inherent to this new focus was a new definition of providers.

Under the earlier legislation, only medical practitioners were covered. With the Canada Health Act, the definition was changed to health care practitioners as a means of expanding the kinds of care covered in the notion of health. Here Minister Bégin was responding to pressure from nurses and others who argued both that they could do much of what doctors did and that their approach was much more in keeping with a focus on health promotion. Future improvements, according to the Act, would require "the cooperative partnership of governments, health professionals, voluntary organizations and individual Canadians."[29]

Health, not merely illness, was established as a public concern. While the previous legislation had said nothing about overall health policy, the new Act stated:

The primary objective of Canadian health care policy is to protect, promote and restore the physical and mental well-being of residents of Canada and to facilitate reasonable access to health services without financial or other barriers.[30]

Similarly, the Preamble emphasized seeking further improvements to health through

combining individual lifestyles that emphasize fitness, prevention of diseases and health promotion with collective action against social, environmental and occupational causes of disease[31]

at the same time as it praised the existing system for treating sickness and disability.

After nearly a quarter century of experience with public health care, Canadians knew what worked and what they wanted. They wanted their public system and they wanted it protected from erosion through charges to individuals. The Canada Health Act was, above all, a reflection of this commitment on the part of Canadians to a universal health system based on need, not money. They recognized the shared risk of ill health. They also recognized that the most efficient and effective way to deal with this risk was to share the responsibility through a public payment scheme.

Lessons on Achieving a Public Health Care System

1. It is possible to develop a universal health system that covers everyone for necessary care.

2. A public system can remove financial barriers to health care.

3. A public insurance scheme does not necessarily mean that governments provide the services or control the institutions directly.

4. With public insurance, hospitals can secure stable financing.

5. Doctors can retain their right to diagnose and treat on the basis of the needs of patients rather than cost.

6. Doctors need not suffer financially, either. Indeed, their security, income, and conditions of work may improve.

7. A public plan can be based on simple legislation that establishes principles without demanding uniformity.

8. A federal scheme can still allow local choices.

9. Opposition can be organized, powerful and recurring, but it can also be countered.

10. Public support grows through experience with a plan that works.

11. The task of providing a universal scheme for accessible, high-quality, cost-effective health care is never completed, but rather must be seen as a process evolving in response to new needs and possibilities.

12. A public scheme is cheaper.

3
Getting Access

When Alice Armstrong was told by her doctor in Ottawa that she had ovarian cancer, she called her sister in Iowa. Her sister's first response was to put a substantial check in the mail. That check said volumes about the difference between health care in Canada and in the United States.

Alice was a professional with a well-paying job in Ottawa. So was her husband, and their children were no longer financially dependent. Her sister's check was not, then, about helping a poor relation. It was about a health care system that determines access on the ability to pay. And in the U.S. even the most economically secure may find they are unable to pay for complicated or lengthy care. In fact, even "Superman" Christopher Reeves has had trouble paying for the care required after he fell from his horse! One study found that nearly 64 million had no health insurance for at least one month during a three-year period, and most with health insurance still have to worry about deductibles and the limits to insurance coverage.[1] Everyone who hears a cancer diagnosis fears for their life. In Canada, though, a cancer diagnosis does not also mean fear of financial hardship. The system is set up to ensure that "no financial barrier should hinder access to care."[2]

There is no question that medicare gave all Canadians universal health insurance. This feature of the system, at least, has never been questioned by its critics. Many have suggested, however, that universal coverage does not necessarily mean universal care, or good care.[3] Cov-

33

erage, whether by private or public insurance, does not always guarantee access to adequate, high-quality health services.

Recognizing this, the Canada Health Act clearly states that accessibility is a basic condition for the federal funding of health care. Such accessibility, according to the Act, means much more than simply getting in to a doctor or hospital sometime, somewhere. Access has a number of components.

First, it means that necessary services must be provided in a way that "does not impede or preclude, either directly or indirectly" access to care. Charges for services constitute one kind of impediment to "reasonable access" that is explicitly forbidden under the Act. But other kinds of impediment are also included in the more general prohibition.

Second, it means that all insured services are provided "on uniform terms and conditions." In other words, there cannot be one service for the rich and one for the poor, one for those who can pay and one for the rest. This system has one tier, caring with the same range and type of services for whomever has medical need.

Third, it means that hospitals and doctors must receive "reasonable compensation for all insured services rendered." The Act thus explicitly acknowledges that providers deserve and need adequate financial reward. Equally important, it recognizes that quality care is most likely to be provided when fair compensation is readily available.[4]

So what does this mean in practice? Have Canadians been getting full access to health care with their public health insurance plan? These questions are best answered by looking at each aspect of access in turn, and by doing so in relation to the situation in the United States.

What Services Do Canadians Get?

One impediment to care is a lack of required services. For hospitals and doctors to be accessible, there must be enough of them to meet medical needs. The founders of Canadian medicare and the people who were pressing the government for action were well aware of this link.

Here, too, the federal government used its money as an incentive to encourage investment in both building hospitals and expanding professional training. Indeed, it saw support of this kind as a first step to developing a national health care scheme. For their part, in the face of postwar shortages, provincial governments could not resist the offer of matching federal grants for hospital construction and similar support for professional training. The result was an enormous growth in both areas. The grants, first offered just after the Second World War, had an obvious impact.

Hospitals

Over the next twenty years, the number of hospital beds available increased by over 100 percent. In spite of massive population growth in the immediate postwar years, the number of beds per person increased by almost 20 percent.[5] This government money for building did not necessarily mean government ownership. For the most part, the new or expanded and improved hospitals remained in the hands of non-profit, non-government organizations.

More beds meant more use. More use meant more expenditures for care on the part of individuals. Both helped create the pressure that resulted in the introduction of the public hospital insurance plan. By 1960, Canadians had many more hospitals than they had had at the end of the war, and those entering the hospital did not have to pay for the service.

The difference was not only obvious in Canada. It was also obvious in comparison with the United States. By 1960, admission rates in Canadian inpatient institutions were higher than those in the United States. Although just under 14 percent of Americans were admitted that year, this was the case for 15 percent of Canadians.[6] Thirty years later, Canadians still enjoyed better access than did their American counterparts. Canada had significantly more hospital beds for their population than was the case in the United States. While there were 6.7 beds for every thousand Canadians in 1989, there were only 5 beds for every thousand Americans.

Not surprisingly, given the greater capacity, more Canadians were admitted to hospital. They also stayed substantially longer than in the United States, with Canadians averaging over three days more in care.

As a result, Canadian hospitals have a higher occupancy rate. Nevertheless, Americans still spent more per person on hospital services.[7]

Given the size of the country, the fact that Canada spends less than does the United States on hospital care yet provides more access to this care is remarkable. Canada is huge, second only to Russia in terms of physical size, but has a very small population. At about 30 million, Canada has fewer people than does California. Although much of the population is huddled along the American border, there are people in need of medical services scattered throughout this enormous country. Based on a practice of pooling resources, many small communities acquired or further developed hospitals with government financial help. So did many smaller provinces. Where hospitals were impractical, nursing stations supported by air transport were supplied. Government intervention did not ensure perfect distribution, but it did go a long way to ensuring that most people who needed hospital services had access to them.

Doctors

The economic incentive worked just as well in terms of expanding the number of health care providers as it did in expanding hospitals. Provinces invested more in educating physicians, nurses, and other health care professionals. At the same time, public hospital insurance meant that these institutions had the secure funding they needed to hire more providers. Public medical insurance guaranteed new doctors both employment and payment.

Between 1960 and 1990, the number of doctors per person in Canada nearly doubled. By 1990 there was one practicing physician for every 448 people. This ratio differed little from that in the United States, where there was a practising physician for every 432 people. The Canadian doctors saw more patients, however. The average number of physician contacts per person that year was 6.9, compared to 5.5 in the United States. As a result, Canadians were more likely to have access to a doctor's care. A recent U.S. study concluded that this was particularly the case for the elderly.[8] Another U.S. study found that much higher fees in the United States were responsible for the facts that

Americans spend 72 percent more per capita on doctors while seeing them less frequently.[9]

What kind of doctors provided this care? The public medical insurance plan was intended to guarantee access to all doctors, general practitioners and specialists alike. And as the public system expanded, so did the number of specialists. By 1990, just over 40 percent of the doctors in Canada were specialists. Here there is a significant difference between the two countries. The ratio of specialist to generalist in Canada is the reverse of that in the United States.[10] While 60 percent of American doctors are specialists, 60 percent of Canadian doctors are in general practice.

This difference does not necessarily mean Americans have better access to specialist care, nor that all these specialists are needed to provide good care. The fact that 10 percent of American medical residents in pathology and plastic surgery failed to find full-time work in 1994 while others failed to find work in their areas of specialization suggest there is an oversupply in some specialties.[11] In Canada, all specialists who want full-time jobs get them and therefore are available to provide care. Moreover, the predominance of specialists in the United States may be at least as much a reflection of the higher incomes that accompany this work as it is a reflection of the medical needs of patients.[12] Indeed, health policy analysts on both sides of the border have argued that we need more emphasis on the kinds of primary care provided by general practitioners. Such care can mean more attention paid to health promotion and disease prevention, in the process both improving health and lowering overall costs to the system.

There can be no doubt that public medical insurance has improved access to doctors. A study on the impact of medical insurance found increased use of doctors by patients "with common and important medical symptoms."[13] Access to Canadian doctors became distributed more on the basis of medical need than on ability to pay.

Although improvement in the distribution of hospitals helped attract doctors to areas outside the urban centers, shortages still persist in some rural areas.[14] This can be partly explained by the fact that doctors have had free choice in terms of where to locate and they have been guaranteed payment wherever they settled. Although it might be assumed that U.S. doctors operating in a primarily private system have more choice about where to locate, this is not necessarily the case. A 1994 report on medical residents found that most job offers came from outside major urban centres. "Fargo, New Mexico, small towns in the West, that's where you have to be willing to go," at least according to one anesthesiologist who had sent out more than 150 resumes.[15]

Nurses

Of course, doctors do not provide most of health care. Because nurses form the overwhelming majority of care providers in both countries, their distribution is at least as important to access as is the distribution of doctors. With government support, both training and nursing centers expanded rapidly in Canada.

The number of registered nurses increased almost threefold between 1960 and 1990. This left Canadians with much better access to nursing care than their U.S. counterparts. In fact, there was a 25 percent difference in the number of nurses per capita, with Canada far in the lead.[16] After doctors, nurses are the most highly trained of care providers and thus their relative numbers can have an important impact on the quality of care.

Overall, the United States has more staff employed in hospitals than is the case in Canada. When full-time equivalents are compared, the United States has significantly more staff in relation to occupied beds.[17] The gap does not necessarily mean that patients receive more or better care, however. It may be largely explained by the greater numbers of administrative staff required to record cost and bill patients. As we shall see in chapter 6, no itemized billing is required in Canada because the patients are not individually charged, and thus a whole array of administrative personnel is absent from Canadian hospitals. Moreover, U.S. hospitals rely particularly heavily on health aides and assistants, the least trained of nursing staff. As a result, patients in American hospitals may be receiving less skilled care.[18]

Non-Hospital Care

Although the Canada Health Act primarily applied to hospitals and doctors, it was also intended to cover extended health care services. According to the Act, these included:

1) nursing home intermediate care service
2) adult residential service
3) home care service
4) ambulatory care service.

The first two categories are mainly about care for the elderly. As is the case with hospitals, the majority of nursing homes and homes for the aged in Canada are nonprofit institutions. And like hospitals, they vary enormously in size. Although a higher proportion of them are operated on a for-profit basis, it was still the case that in 1990 less than 30 percent of the beds were offered in for-profit institutions.[19] Nevertheless, most of the money for such facilities comes from the public purse, regardless of ownership.

This public sponsorship helps explain why Canada has so many more nursing home beds than is the case in the United States. With one bed for every 113 persons, Canada has over four and a half times as many beds, proportionately, as does the United States, where there is a nursing home bed for one out of every 523 citizens.[20]

Canada also has residential care facilities for the physically handicapped, the developmentally delayed, and the psychiatrically disabled. More than 80 percent of the facilities for the developmentally delayed and the physically handicapped are nonprofit institutions that receive substantially government funding. For-profit care is more common for the psychiatrically disabled, but most of these facilities also receive significant government subsidies.[21]

Care for those who live outside institutions is both more variable and more difficult to track. As with nursing homes, the home care services paid for by public funds may be provided by government, by nonprofit agencies, or by for-profit firms. For-profit firms are a small part of the picture, however, and are virtually nonexistent in many areas of the country.

What is included in the services paid for through the public plan varies across the country as well. Usually, the services include home nursing and various therapies. Non-medical services such as housekeeping, house maintenance, respite care, and meal preparation are also common. Medical supplies and devices are frequently provided, as are some prescription drugs. Although the elderly on both sides of the border are eligible for publicly supported care, one 1996 study found that "Canadian elderly receive four times as many home or nursing home visits as American elderly."[22] While most of those receiving care are over age sixty-five, a significant proportion are from other age groups.[23] These services provided outside institutions may be long-term for those with chronic problems or disabilities.[24]

The Canada Health Act was extended to ambulatory services as a means of encouraging alternatives to inpatient care. Outpatient care was thought to not only be cheaper and preferred by those using the services but also more in keeping with a new focus on health promotion and community care. Although hospitals had been providing outpatient services, there was a further incentive to do so when the federal government offered financial help that extended beyond inpatient care.

Similarly, some provinces had community clinics and community health centers before medicare and the extension of funding was an important factor leading to a new interest in these kinds of services. In Ontario, for example, there were health centers very much like the Health Maintenance Organizations (HMOs) familiar to Americans through such organizations as Kaiser Permanente. The medical establishment opposed these centers with their salaried providers in group practices. Yet a study of one such center found that "although the group practice had no financial incentive to economize on inpatient care, its rate of hospitalization was lower by about a quarter." There seemed to be a greater emphasis on health promotion, combined with a higher utilization of testing services.[25] One of these centers had been started by the steelworkers' union but government funding was eventually forthcoming. As has been the case with other centers in the province, funding was offered in the form of either per capita or global grants. Whatever the funding formula for the centers, patients could still choose if and when to use them. Their medical cards or numbers enrolled them in the public health care system, not exclusively in a particular center.

The province of Quebec went farther than other jurisdictions in developing a combination of health and community service centers. These CLSCs (*centres locaux de services communitaires*, or local community service centers) were intended to provide the main entrance to the entire array of public health and community services. Staffed by salaried, multidisciplinary teams, they were intended to integrate services at the community level. With health defined in very broad terms to include economic and social as well as biological aspects, these centers were designed to not only treat problems but also promote health. Like the centers in Ontario, however, they met with strong opposition from physicians committed to fee-for-service practice. In response to the Quebec initiative, the physicians set up their own group practices and tried to compete with the CLSCs by offering twenty-four-hour reception services. Although the CLSCs are more common in poor and rural areas, 159 centers can be found throughout Quebec. And although they do not all provide the full array of services or the main entrance to other kinds of health services, they do offer many communities an alternative to physician-centered care. A study completed twenty years after medicare began in Quebec concluded that these centers were "more community oriented, nearer to holistic medicine, tied in with the psychosocial components of basic primary care, more attentive to complex problems such as family violence, mental health, sexual abuse."[26]

Although community clinics have received support from governments and communities, they are still strongly resisted by doctors. This is partly explained by the guaranteed fee-for-service payment from public funds. The 1990 study found that less than 3 percent of physicians worked in community health clinics, health service organizations, or CLSCs. The researchers concluded that "there have been fewer incentives in Canada to explore alternatives to traditional solo practice than exist in the competitive medical marketplace of the United States."[27]

In addition to community health centers, government money also goes to walk-in clinics. These have been growing in number in Canada and are seen by some as a substitute for emergency care in hospitals, both because they are often located near where people are employed and because they often have long operating hours. The doctors who work in these clinics still bill the government on a fee-for-service basis but many do not actually receive this income. Instead, the money goes to the for-profit company that organizes the clinic and handles the administration, including the doctors' salaries. The patients who use these centers do what they do in any doctor's office. They simply provide their health care card or number and there is no restriction on use.

Rehabilitation hospitals also provide services for outpatients. Like other hospitals, their basic budgets come from government sources. However, a higher proportion of these hospitals are for-profit and many of these offer services in addition to those covered by the public health insurance plan. In the case of these additional services, the hospitals can charge fees to patients.

Many of those who use rehabilitation services have work-related injuries and thus are covered by workers' compensation. In Canada, these are provincial programs that vary across the country. For the most part, the medical needs of those with claims are automatically covered by medicare, although extra services may be covered by workers' compensation with a view to speeding up recovery time. Rehabilitation services in particular may be paid for by workers' compensation. Because there is a national health insurance plan, however, workers' compensation in Canada is more about income replacement than it is about medical care. This contrasts sharply with workers' compensation in the United States. When American chemical workers visited Canada to view the health care system firsthand, the issue of workers' compensation was raised by a man with personal experience. Injured at work, he was placed on workers' compensation coverage. Injured at home while on workers' compensation, he could not have his fractured hip covered by his workplace insurance. Workers' compensation would not pay the health bills because it was not a workplace injury. This would not happen in Canada because the hip injury in either location would be covered by public insurance.

Problems related to getting to the hospital or doctor can also restrict access. Various kinds of transportation services are offered by governments. Ambulance services are provided in almost all jurisdictions, and may be operated by the government or by for-profit firms. Similarly, transportation is available in many areas for the disabled or the elderly who need help getting to health care services.

Fees

With more hospitals, doctors, nursing homes and homecare services, care became more accessible. But access is also related to what the individual must pay at the point of service, as the Canada Health Act recognized. For some, fees of any sort can limit access to essential care.

Therefore, according to the Act, medical practitioners are not allowed to extra-bill; that is, to charge their patients more than the rate the doctors collectively negotiate with the government. Nor can hospitals charge user fees to patients for basic services. The only exception applies to those with chronic illnesses that make them more or less permanent residents of care institutions. In such cases, some charges for meals or accommodation are permitted.

This is not to suggest that the issue of fees has been settled once and for all in Canada. In spite of the fact that the idea of user fees has been examined and rejected on the basis of the evidence, there is always some group or other suggesting that fees will solve whatever the current problem with health care use or delivery. As health economist Robert Evans and his colleagues put it, "Like zombies in the night, these ideas may be intellectually dead but are never buried."[28] The zombies keep reappearing, they argue, both because there are well-organized groups who have much to gain from such fees and because user charges seem to make common sense to many people. At the same time, those demanding fees have seldom prevailed both because there is very strong support for the current fee-less system and because the evidence challenges the claims of those demanding fees.

The arguments, the defenders, and the evidence about user fees are very similar in Canada and the United States. The most common argument on both sides of the border is that user fees will ensure appropriate use of services. There are several commonsense assumptions behind this argument. One is that people will think twice about going to a doctor or hospital if they have to pay for some of the care. This is connected to a second notion, namely that people currently misuse services that are without fees. Another basis for this idea that fees will ensure appropriate use is that people appreciate a service more if they have to pay for it. In other words, it's not the money, it's the principles. The principles are that people value more what they have to pay for and that nothing should be free.

Yet the facts do not support this commonsense notion that fees will prevent abuse and allocate care to those who truly need it. Perhaps the most important fact refuting this notion is that most care is not initiated by the patient. While it is true that patients often take the first step by calling a doctor, most of the rest in the chain of care is determined by doctors. Patients cannot simply approach a hospital and ask for a hysterectomy, for example. In Canada, less than 15 percent of the money spent on physicians can be attributed to direct visits to primary physicians, and some of these are return visits recommended by the doctor in question. As a group of researchers who carefully examined these claims put it, "If nearly ninety per cent of medicare expenditures are thus a consequence of an explicit physician admission and referral, and some undetermined portion of the rest are initiated by the practitioner, this does not leave a lot of scope for savings by reducing *patient-initiated* 'frivolous' demands."[29] That doctors, rather than patients, determine most use may help explain why "all the evidence indicates that in-patient use is insensitive to patient charges."[30]

When patients do ask for services, there is no evidence that many of them do so frivolously. Even if a doctor determines that a patient who visits the office or the emergency room has no treatable complaint, this does not prove that the call was frivolous. A patient may be seeking advice for what turns out to be simply a bad cough that will cure itself in time, but the bad cough could well be pneumonia. Only the physician, and in some situations the nurse, can tell for sure, and if pneumonia is detected early, both costs and suffering may be greatly reduced.

Instead of ensuring more appropriate use, fees may allow frivolous use by the rich while discouraging necessary use by the poor. Fees cannot be expected to improve the use patterns of the rich, for they are unlikely to be deterred by extra charges when deciding whether to use health services. Further, if extra charges ensure a place at the front of the line, such charges may encourage some extra use on the part of those who can afford the fees. Meanwhile, the poor may decide that they have to go without needed care. A study conducted in the United States concluded that coinsurance charges "reduced the demand for care in situations where care was likely to be highly effective as much as it did in situations where care was deemed to be only rarely effective."[31]

Fees do not work to appropriately allocate care primarily because the "laws" of supply and demand do not work here. The theory of supply and demand rests on the assumption of readily available choices, alternatives, and information. For the most part, people do not have a choice about when, if, where, or how to get sick or become disabled. This is especially the case for the most expensive health care services such as those brought into play after a car accident or a breast cancer diagnosis. Few are in a position to shop around, and if they are, seldom have the expertise required to make the appropriate choice. Moreover, no one can easily know what they are shopping for, given that they cannot predict with any accuracy what illnesses or accidents will hit them. When they do become ill, choosing whether or not to seek treatment may mean a choice between life and death or between recovery and permanent disability. And it is often a choice that has to be made quickly or while incapacitated.

Given the nature of health care needs, what extra fees mainly do is make the sick pay even when they have no choice about being ill. Research in the province of Saskatchewan found that fees did not lead to better use of health services. Instead, their effect "is simply to transfer costs from the public to the private budget with the burden of such transfers falling disproportionately on the sicker members of the population."[32] Given that the poor are more likely to be ill, the burden of payment falls disproportionately on them.

Clearly, then, user fees do not result in more appropriate use of services. And free services do not necessarily mean that people value them less. Indeed, as we have seen, Canadians place a very high value on their free health care system. While these facts may be conceded by proponents of extra fees, there are still many on both sides of the border who argue that user fees are necessary to bring more money into the system. In both countries, doctors and policy makers have maintained that fees will put more money into care and thus improve overall services.

Obviously, if patients pay additional money to receive services, then there will be more money in the system. But this will be the case only if three conditions apply. First, the number of people using the system will have to at least remain the same. Second, the cost of collecting the fees must be less than the amount collected. And third, the money has to be spread around within the system if it is to improve overall services. None of these conditions necessarily apply.

Fees can discourage use, and thus the overall amount coming into the system may decline. Furthermore, if fees discourage people from seeking treatment until their problems become very severe, the long term costs of care may increase for the individual and for the services. An Ontario study found that the poor did just that when fees were in place.[33]

The cost of collecting fees can significantly reduce the overall financial gain. Additional administrative costs are involved. This is particularly the case if fee collection requires a distinction to be made between those who can afford the fee and those who cannot. In the United States, proponents of fees sometimes argue that no one will be charged or denied service because they cannot pay but it is not clear on what basis this distinction will be made, who will make it and what it will cost to make.[34] In Canada, those making policy have been convinced more than once by the evidence that the financial benefits of fees are more than offset by the resulting disparity and additional costs of administration.

Doctors have been less convinced. Fees can mean they make more money. When doctors in Canada extra-billed, the money went directly to them, so perhaps it is not surprising that they saw extra-billing as putting more money into health care. But the system as a whole saw little benefit. While doctors also argued that such extra billing was essential to professional autonomy and the integrity of the doctor–patient relationship, they were never able to successfully explain why paying some additional cash creates autonomy or ensures integrity. As Tommy Douglas put it, "When someone says 'It's not the money, it's the principle' you can be sure it's the money."[35]

Fees may not get equally distributed throughout the system but they do make a difference in access. Canada forbids fees for basic services. And there are no deductibles or co–insurance payments. Contrast this to the $760 deductible for the first 60 days of coverage under U.S. Medicare; $190 co–insurance for the 61st through the 90th day; the $380 per day after the 91st day but coverage in any benefit period is limited to the number of lifetime reserve days available; the $95 per day for the 21st through the 100th day per benefit period and the $311 hospital insurance premium.[36] As a result, only 0.7 percent of Canadians report that financial barriers prevented them from getting necessary care. According to a study on utilization in Newfoundland between 1992 and 1995, "Both the probability of being hospitalized and the utilization of general practitioners is higher for groups with lower socio-economic status; the elimination of financial barriers is allowing individuals with lower socio-economic status to access services according to need (real or perceived)."[37] In contrast, 7 percent of Americans say financial barriers meant they were unable to get required care. Other barriers to access remain in Canada, such as location or time arrangements for services. But even in terms of these barriers, Canadians are significantly better off than Americans. Only 3 percent of Canadians blamed nonfinancial barriers for their inability to get care while this was the case for 6 percent of Americans.[38]

Reasonable Compensation: What Providers Are Paid

With all the talk about extra fees, it would be easy to think that public insurance means low incomes for doctors. But this is simply not the case. The Canada Health Act requires that medical practitioners receive reasonable compensation. The fact that they are second only to judges and magistrates in terms of income clearly demonstrates that this is indeed the case.

Almost all Canada's doctors work on a fee-for-service basis. The fees are not set by the federal government, or any other government for that matter. They are negotiated by the doctors' associations with provincial governments, with different fees established for different procedures and treatments. Doctors have proven to be very powerful in this process.

The development of the fee schedule in the province of Ontario, for example, was once described as the government wrestling the doctors to the ceiling. This kind of bargaining outcome was evident in the most recent negotiations in that province. The Ontario Medical Association won an increase of 1.5 percent compounded annually in the total fee-for-service billings and a price increase of 2.25 percent in the second year of the three-year contract. The agreement guarantees that there will be no reductions over this three-year period. All this is built on a foundation of what the doctors billed the system in the previous year, which turns out to be as much as 8 percent more than they were supposed to bill. The enforcement mechanism in the previous agreement to prevent over-billing was dropped and not replaced. Doctors were also offered the option of going on salary or converting to a capitation formula, one that would pay them a fixed sum for every regular patient. In addition, the government promised to increase their contributions to the payment of malpractice insurance by a maximum of $34 million. It is common for provincial governments in Canada to subsidize heavily the medical malpractice insurance premiums of the doctors within their jurisdictions.[39] In contrast, American doctors spend about 4 percent of their income on malpractice insurance—an amount that would almost make up the income differences in the two countries. Moreover, American doctors are much more likely to be sued for malpractice, in part because many patient costs are not covered by insurance.[40]

In this public system, then, doctors' incomes are primarily determined by three things: the negotiated fee schedule, the patients they serve, and the hours they work. These factors necessarily result in some differences in doctors' incomes, within and among provinces. It is safe to say, however, that all Canadian doctors have incomes that are well above average and some do much better than that. When Ontario attempted to cap doctors' gross income at about $C 400,000, there were howls of outrage from the profession. Clearly not all doctors earned more than the just over $100,000 given as the average.[41]

More than one doctor has threatened to leave Canada for what are seen as the greener fields in the United States. At first glance, it looks like doctors there are significantly better off when it comes to income. Figures for 1989 show self-employed doctors in the United States earning 25 percent more than their Canadian colleagues. But a number of things must be taken into account before any such conclusion can be drawn.

First, these figures only include the self-employed. While in Canada this would cover almost all doctors, in the United States the many salaried doctors would be excluded. And salaried doctors are likely to earn less than those who are self-employed. Second, there are significantly more specialists in the United States, and specialists too are likely to earn more money. Third, income is more evenly distributed among doctors in Canada than is the case in the United States. As a result, many more doctors in Canada are likely to earn at least the average income while this is not likely to be the case in the United States. One U.S. study found that pediatricans paid according to the 1992 Medicare fee schedule would earn $35,000 a year compared to $241,000 for thoracic surgeons.[42] Although a Canadian thoracic surgeon might well earn $241,000, it would be very difficult for a Canadian pediatrician to earn that little. Moreover, a Canadian doctor's income is quite stable, given that the government guarantees payment, while an American doctor's income may vary depending on how good insurance companies and patients are about paying their bills.

Average and national data can hide quite wide income differences among doctors, especially in the United States, where the disparities are wider. They also make it difficult to get a clear picture of what any particular doctor really earns. Specific cases from both countries help make the real earnings picture more concrete, although they cannot capture the range of medical incomes.

Take the case of an Ontario physician, for example. One of forty-one obstetricians practicing in Ottawa (population about 700,000), Dr. Warren Harrison delivers about 200 babies a year. In 1995, he billed his provincial insurance plan $213,500. He also provided extra services for the military and for diplomats living in the nation's capital. And he saw patients from the neighbouring province of Quebec. For these services, he billed other governments an additional $42,000 for a total of $255,500 from public insurance plans. His total billings would have amounted to roughly $270,000, but an agreement the doctors had made with the provencial government reduced this by an estimated $15,000. If doctors collectively had kept within their promised total billing range, no deduction would have been made to Dr. Harrison's charges for the insurance plan.

Of course, not all the money goes into Dr. Harrison's pocket. In 1995, obstetricians paid $4,900 in malpractice insurance, with Ontario public insurance picking up the rest of the $18,000 premium. He also paid close to $50,000 in wages and benefits for his secretary and part-time nurse. Rent, office supplies, property taxes, and utilities consumed just over $36,000. Another $10,000 went for accounting services and bank charges, depreciation and insurance, equipment, and cleaning. Just over $90,000 of his $255,500, then, was allocated to these necessary expenses.

In addition, Dr. Harrison's memberships in professional organizations cost him $1,900, he spent $2,500 to attend a conference in Mexico, and was able to write off $4,100 on the business use of his car. He thus spent 43 percent of his gross income on expenses, leaving him with $144,400 before personal taxes. After taxes, he was left with $88,800, of which he spent $14,900 on disability insurance and a private pension plan (although he is already collecting $40,000 in a military pension), leaving him with $73,900 in disposable income from his current practice. Since 1995, his fee schedule as on obstetrician has gone up by 30 percent, and the provincial clawback mechanism has been eliminated.

Although obstetricians are better paid than general practitioners, they are among the lowest paid of the specialists in Ontario, lower than internists, for example. And they have "onerous on-call responsibilities," in the words of the Society of Obstetricians and Gynecologists of Canada. As the spokesperson for Ottawa's obstetricians in a dispute with the provincial government over the fee schedule, Dr. Harrison clearly felt he was underpaid, and that the readers of Ottawa's daily newspaper would agree with him once they learned the details of his annual income and expenses.[43]

Yet compare his case with the following example from the United States. Dr. Claudia Fegan reports that, in her busy internal medicine practice in Chicago, consisting of six internists, her income is derived from a measure of her "productivity," minus the expenses required to keep the practice in operation. As in Ottawa, these overhead expenses include staff salaries, office space rental, equipment purchases, answering service, computer software, and so on. From each physician's productivity, or revenue generated, the percentage required to pay the overhead is deducted. In bad years that has been as much as 73 percent of each physician's productivity, and in good years as little as 55 percent. For example, a busy physician in Dr. Fegan's practice seeing 300 to 400 patients a month might generate $390,000 in a year. This would result in a gross income of $175,000, from which would be deducted the physician-specific expenses, such as health insurance premiums, disability premiums, and federal taxes.

A more common practice among small groups of physicians in the United States is for the more senior partners to pay a lower percentage of the overhead and for the more junior partners to take home less of the revenue they generate. Finally, some groups just charge all of the partners a flat fee to run the office, regardless of the revenue they generate, thus extracting a higher percentage from partners who are less busy and generate less revenue. With the cumbersome billing structures U.S. physicians confront, regardless of their method of meeting office expenses, they take home less of their generated revenue than their northern neighbors. And, in the end, they may make little more than their Canadian counterparts, even when their expenses are equitably shared.

In general, a negotiated fee schedule for a universal program allows a range of salaries and high incomes for doctors at the same time as it limits gross disparities. One fee schedule within each Canadian jurisdiction also means that wages are unlikely to vary as significantly by sex and race. There are differences in male and female doctors' incomes, but this primarily reflects differences in hours of work and areas of specialization. In Canada, male physicians had yearly incomes 52 percent higher than the women practicing medicine. In the United States, the median weekly earnings for male physicians in 1996 were 72 percent higher than that for female physicians.[44] The greater uniformity in Canadian fees may help explain why, in 1990, 27 percent of Canadian doctors were female, compared to 17 percent in the United States.[45]

The requirement in the Canada Health Act for reasonable compensation does not extend to other health care providers. However, the expansion of facilities and the stable financing did help the mainly female workers who provide most of health care. Before medicare, most health care work was done by nurses training or trained in a hospital and paid as if they were working for love, not money. By the 1990s, nursing education happened in colleges or universities and nurses in training no longer provided free care. Four out of five of them belonged to a union that had won decent wages, employment security, and significant benefits. In some provinces, these wages were negotiated at the provincial level, resulting in a uniform wage structure for nurses. For the most part, nurses were employees of individual institutions. The central bargaining helped equalize employment opportunities for nurses across a province at the same time as it helped employers recruit in an organized manner.

Uniform Terms and Conditions: One-Tier Care

When Alice Armstrong's doctor decided she needed radiation treatment, she was sent to the Ottawa Civic Hospital. The decision was based on the facilities available there. If the diagnosis had been given to a dirty, penniless man waiting in line for a welfare check, the doctor is very likely to send him to Ottawa Civic as well. Indeed, the man could easily end up in the private room next door to Alice. This is what the Canada Health Act means by uniform terms and conditions.

One way Canada tries to ensure that services are provided under uniform terms and conditions to both Alice and the welfare recipient is by forbidding private insurance coverage of those services covered by the public plan. No one has the choice of purchasing insurance for special care in Canada if the services are available under the public plan. You cannot, for example, buy private insurance to cover basic hospital services. Nor can private insurance companies offer plans that cover the services of a cardiac surgeon.

The other way Canada tries to ensure uniform terms and conditions is by providing the same basic services in every institution. There are few if any visible differences between services provided in wealthy and poor neighborhoods. There are differences among hospitals in terms of specialties and the range of services. So, for example, in Toronto the Orthopedic and Arthritic hospital specializes in hip and knee replacement, and the Princess Margaret Hospital treats cancer patients. Children's hospitals are also available to serve the specific needs of that population but the hospital is open to any child, as are the services within it.

As a result, patients and doctors select services primarily on the basis of location and specialty, on the basis of doctors they like or treatments available rather than on the basis of their membership in particular insurance schemes. Unlike the United States, where a Harvard professor says she has a fine health care plan as long as she gets sick within a mile of Harvard Square, hospitals such as the one in Montreal serve children from throughout the province and even from throughout the country, without regard to any private insurance conditions.

Within hospitals, there are no public and private wards. The most common kind of hospital room has two beds separated by curtains and a bathroom for the use of those two patients. There are rooms for four patients, and rooms with more beds are sometimes found in children's hospitals in particular. Private rooms exist, but the doctor could well decide that the only private room available is needed more by the welfare recipient than by Alice. If the doctor makes this decision, then there is no charge to the patient. If the patient makes this decision, then there will be a charge to the patient or their insurance scheme.

Similarly, there are no distinctions within the system in terms of levels of care or kinds of medical services available made on the basis of differences in insurance schemes. If a special bed is required for a person with a back injury, the bed will be supplied without regard to any insurance scheme. If a choice is to be made between surgery or drugs, the decisions is based on what the doctor and patient decide is the best option, not on the basis of what an insurance scheme will cover. If Alice has to choose between chemotherapy and radiation, it is a choice that has no direct financial consequences for her and the welfare recipient has the same alternatives. And the drugs they receive in the hospital will be the same, as will their length of stay.

Why not make the rich pay and offer them the option of seeking other care? One reason follows from the belief that care should be based on need, not money, on diagnosis rather than ability to pay. In general, people do not get ill by choice, nor do they choose their illnesses. Extra effort may help people stay healthy and avoid risks but many medical problems are beyond individual control. To base the quality of care on money is similar to denying care on the basis of money. It is simply unfair not only to the poor but also to the more affluent who would may find lengthy and complicated illnesses difficult to finance in spite of their more secure economic position.

Another reason is that if everyone has to use the same system, they have the same interest in making sure that system is good. If Alice has the room next door to the welfare recipient and sees the same radiologist, she has every reason to want both the room and the doctor to be good, for both of them. Allowing those who can afford it to access other services reduces their interest in the overall quality of care provided for others.

Equally important, once care can be purchased, those paying for care may object to the use of their tax money for services they are not using. Or they may at least object to care being provided according to the kinds of standards they are purchasing. The result can be an undermining of the entire funding system. Yet purchased care is heavily subsidized by the infrastructure paid for by tax dollars, and this is the case on both sides of the border. Much of the money that goes into the education of doctors, nurses, and other providers also comes from tax dollars. So does much of the funding for medical research and the medical infrastructure. When individuals pay for care, they are rarely paying the entire cost of their care, even when the bills are high. And there is necessarily an inequality involved, because only the sick use the service, regardless of their incomes.

Allowing the rich to pay for special care can also distort the overall quality of services in terms of what services are provided where. Providing two kinds of care can lead to costly duplication and an expansion of the services covered by private schemes and a reduction in those that are not. Those who pay may assume they should go to the front of the line, in the process perhaps denying care to those who need service more.

Not all differences or all private insurance schemes are eliminated by the uniform terms and conditions requirement. The public scheme applies to those services defined as essential. Plastic surgery carried out to remove wrinkles or for other purposes defined as nonessential to health, for example, or surgery done to remove tattoos may not be covered under the public plan. In such instances, private insurance coverage is quite possible. Alternative therapies provided by massage therapists and others are unlikely to be offered in the public system, although the services of chiropractors and physiotherapists often are. In the case of physiotherapy and chiropractic, however, additional services from these providers could still be covered under a private scheme. Ontario is one province that allows a limited number of visits to chiropractors to be paid for by public insurance. Additional coverage can be purchased from private insurers. Similarly, hospital services such as in-room televison sets and telephones may not be part of all provincial insurance schemes, although any essentials like soap and toothpaste, drugs, and tests are part of the public plan.

Waiting Lists

Access is not just about whether or not there are facilities but also about how long people have to wait for care. All countries ration services one way or another. In Canada, this rationing does not depend on ability to pay. The media on both sides of the border have suggested that rationing instead takes the form of long waiting lines for care. While they cannot deny that Alice and the welfare recipient might have an equal chance at care, they do claim that both of them may have to wait too long for care.

Canadians do not wait for care that is required immediately. Alice had her surgery booked in the doctor's office while she was assimilating the news of her diagnosis. Emergency rooms are readily available in all urban centers, and all patients urgently requiring care can be admitted without regard to ability to pay, health care plan, or place of residence. In rural areas, ambulances on the road or in the air can deliver patients quickly to emergency centers.

Surgery that is deemed medically necessary on an urgent basis is also done quickly. As a recent survey of the Canadian system put it, "in virtually all cases, Canadians who need emergency or urgent care receive it in a timely fashion; it is extremely uncommon for patients on surgical waiting lists to die." Indeed, there is no evidence that they are more likely to die than their American counterparts. There is, however, evidence to suggest that in the United States "the uninsured receive less trauma-related care and have a higher mortality rate."[46] We can assume no such differences exist in Canada, given that everyone is covered for care.

Comparisons between Canada and the United States do reveal differences in waiting times for some kinds of surgery. In the case of knee replacement surgery, for example, Canadians waited significantly longer than Americans. While waiting for knee surgery may be inconvenient or even painful, it is unlikely to be life-threatening. It is not surprising then that only 15 percent of Canadians felt their waiting time was unacceptable for this surgery.[47] When it comes to general surgery, the research indicates that there is very little difference in the level of patient satisfaction. Nearly 84 percent of Canadian respondents and just over 85 percent of American ones were "very or somewhat satisfied with their waiting times."[48]

In the province of Alberta there has been a great deal of discussion about access to cataract surgery. The response of the Consumers Association of Canada (Alberta) was to conduct a telephone survey in April 1994 of the opthamologist clinics in the major cities of the province. They found that patients in all the cities studied had quite reasonable access to public care. In Calgary and Edmonton, appointments could be made within four weeks with 70 to 80 percent of the surgeons. For those surgeons regularly performing cataract surgery in hospitals, the operation could be arranged with waiting periods of two to five weeks in Calgary and three to eight weeks in Edmonton. In Lethbridge, Medicine Hat, and Red Deer, appointments can be made within one to eight weeks, followed by surgery in five to twenty weeks. None of these waiting periods are excessive for cataract surgery, and all can lead to cost-free care for the patient. In short, there is little support for the claim that public insurance leads to long waiting times or that Canadians wait longer than Americans for care.

Sex, Race, and Culture

Canada is a multicultural and multiracial society. In fact, Toronto has a more diverse population than any other city in the world. Not only does Canada have a varied population, it also has an explicit policy promoting multiculturalism.

This emphasis on difference can be traced back, in large part, to the two national groups responsible for the political founding of Canada. The British North America Act brought together one area dominated by the English and another dominated by the French. Central to this confederation was the maintenance of French culture, primarily through provincial control of health, education, and social programs. From 1867 on, then, it was recognized that Canada would not follow the American lead towards a "melting pot" of culture.

As a result of this compromise, there are a wide variety of health services available in French. This is particularly the case in Quebec, where the official language is French and all services must be available in that language at least. Other provinces such as Ontario, Manitoba, and New Brunswick also provide services in French, although on a more limited and restricted scale. Access is even more limited where the French population is small, as it is in many parts of Canada.

The white European population is the single largest group in Canada, albeit one divided along linguistic lines. After that, no one racial or cultural group predominates in terms of numbers. Aboriginal Peoples are the next largest, but they are themselves quite internally divided into distinct nations and cultural groups. This distribution contrasts with that in the United States, where African American and Hispanic populations are found in significantly large numbers. In some ways, then, cultural and racial diversity takes different forms in Canada. These forms in turn are related to health care services.

In Canada, universality helps ensure access that does not follow racial or cultural lines. In the United States, by contrast, one in five African Americans does not have health insurance,[49] and "those of Hispanic origin had the highest chance of lacking coverage throughout 1995."[50]

Access is much more than coverage, however. As the original French populations who negotiated confederation knew quite well, sensitivity to cultural, racial, and linguistic differences is critical in a service that is as intimate and personal as health care. Canada has done less well in these terms than it has on universality.[51]

This is particularly the case with Aboriginal Peoples. Health care for this quite varied group was left mainly to the federal government by the British North America Act. In recent years more and more responsibility for health care has been transferred to provincial or Aboriginal control. This transfer reflects, in part at least, the recognition that a more culturally sensitive approach is required, one that responds to needs as defined by the Aboriginal People rather than by policy makers in the nation's capital.

The federal government, among other agencies, has supported research demonstrating the poor health status among Aboriginal Peoples.[52] Although much of this poor health can be attributed to nutrition, housing, unemployment, and loss of community, some at least can be related to the way health care has been provided to Aboriginal Peoples. Services have been made available, but the services have too frequently been based on standards and practices developed for the dominant white culture. Such health care delivery often seemed to undermine traditional practices while failing to provide new ones that adapt modern science to Aboriginal culture.

There have long been some services designed by and for Aboriginal Peoples, although these services were scattered and usually unconnected. More recently, however, governments at all levels have begun to respond in concrete ways to the demands from Aboriginal groups for appropriate care. Ontario midwifery provides just one example. When midwifery became a regulated profession in that province, a special procedure was developed to educate and accredit Aboriginal midwives. This process was intended not only to recognize the value of traditional practices but also to acknowledge and credit prior learning experience in Aboriginal communities.

While the public system has been exposed as insensitive, that public system makes it possible to exert pressure for more concerted action on developing culturally appropriate health care delivery. The same could be said for the health services provided to other minority groups in Canada. Because the system was based primarily on the private delivery of care, many of the services have been developed with particular cultures in mind. There are, for instance, a significant number of Jewish hospitals in Canada, along with a fair number of Italian residential-care facilities and special clinics for immigrants. These institutions are eligible for public funding, as long as they have been accredited to provide care.

Similarly, a publicly funded system can plan to change the way providers deliver care. Because universities in Canada are public institutions, which are influenced by public policies on health care, systematic policies on how care providers are educated can be developed. In this way it is possible to encourage culturally sensitive training.

The task of providing culturally, linguistically and racially appropriate access is enormous in a country as diverse as Canada. Language alone can constitute a significant barrier, especially under the distressing circumstances often associated with the delivery of care. Canada certainly still has work to do before all groups have their care provided in ways that are in keeping with their particular needs and traditional practices. Yet Canada's public health insurance system has recognized the problem and initiated some services to address this important, and huge, task.

Although each of these populations requiring special services to meet their needs include women, women as a group share some particular health concerns. More women than men on both sides of the border use the health care system. This higher utilization rate is explained, in large measure, by women's greater longevity and by the attention health providers and researchers have paid to women's reproductive systems.

Although biases remain, women in Canada do have better access to health services than their U.S. counterparts. "In 1995, 73 percent of long-term health care institution residents aged 65 and over were women."[53] All these Canadian women had their care heavily subsidized by the public insurance plan. In the childbearing years, "Americans with Medicaid wait for prenatal care and many Americans receive no prenatal care at all,"[54] while all Canadian women are eligible for prenatal care. Abortions are performed as part of the public health services. And, while access to reproductive technologies varies from province to province, some aspects are covered in every province.

That Canadian women have higher utilization rates than men and better access than American women, does not necessarily mean care is accessible in the sense of responding adequately or appropriately to their needs.[55] Like their American counterparts, Canadian women have been demonstrating both that they have needs particular to their sex and that these needs are not being met by the health care system. Women surveyed by the National Forum on Health objected to the inappropriate use of drugs, technologies and devices, the paternalistic attitudes of providers, the treatment of women and their bodies as machines with parts to be fixed in the shortest possible time, and the particular barriers faced by women with disabilities, women with experiences of abuse or battering, and by women with varied cultural or sexual backgrounds.[56]

This list would sound familiar to most American women. The difference in Canada, though, is that there is a public insurance scheme that could use its financial power to encourage changes that respond to these concerns on a systematic basis. And it has done so in funding women's clinics in hospitals, health promotion services, and centers for research on women's health. Although far from enough, a public system does ensure women access to basic services and some hope for more women-centered care.

Summary

Canadians, then, have an accessible system with plenty of choice for both patients and doctors. As an editorial in the *New England Journal of Medicine* put it, "the Canadian system is probably best characterized by the absence of constraints on the autonomy of patients and clinicians."[57]

4

Comprehensive Coverage

What do Canadians get access to with their universal coverage? It is difficult to challenge the claim that public insurance provides universal coverage for all Canadians. Access may be somewhat more open to question, but the data on the availability of doctors, hospitals, nursing homes, and other services certainly support the argument that the Canadian public system provides access that is at least as good as that in the United States. And there is ample evidence that Canadians face fewer financial barriers to care than do their American neighbors.

According to the Canada Health Act, Canadians not only are entitled to care that is universal and accessible, they also have the right to comprehensive services. So it seems clear that coverage for a broad range of health care requirements is a feature of the Canadian system as well. There is more dispute, however, about the quality of the Canadian public system. And there are claims that the competitive system in the United States provides better care. It is important, then, to look both at what is covered by public insurance and at the quality of the care that is offered in the Canadian health system.

Hospital Coverage

The Canada Health Act defines comprehensiveness to include "all insured health services provided by hospitals."[1] The legislation makes it clear that these services are very broadly defined. They include all inpatient and outpatient services as long as they are "medically necessary." And medical necessity is itself broadly defined to cover all that is required "for the purpose of maintaining health, preventing disease or diagnosing or treating an injury, illness or disability."[2]

The Canada Health Act, like the initial hospital insurance act, makes it clear that health care in hospitals involves much more than treatment and cure. The Act specifically names those things deemed necessary for health care.

I. Basic Needs

The service listed first is the most basic to health, namely, food and housing. Meals and accommodation are to be provided without charge as part of care. While the legislation states that these must at least conform to a minimum standard, it also declares that "preferred accommodation" will be covered as part of the public insurance if it is medically required. In other words, the act requires that a welfare recipient stays in a private ward as part of the standard package if the private ward is necessary to health. This might well be the case if, for example, the patient is at high risk from infection, is in particular need of rest, or is facing imminent death.

II. Diagnosis and Tests

The list also includes all the ways people are tested and examined in hospitals. The Act explicitly refers to laboratory and radiological procedures. But it goes on to add "other diagnostic procedures." Thus, if new means of testing and diagnosing are developed, these too are covered by public insurance when they are performed in a hospital and are medically necessary. Whether a procedure is performed for inpatients or outpatients, Canadians have the right to a full array of services designed to find out what is wrong with them.

III. Treatment

Not surprisingly, all means of treatment are on the list of insured hospital services. The use of the operating room and the case room is part of the package. And anesthetic services are explicitly included as well. Other kinds of less invasive treatment are also covered. Radiotherapy and physiotherapy facilities are explicitly mentioned, indicating that it is not only treatment by a physician that is considered central to necessary care. Canadians need not be concerned about delaying or avoiding required surgery because of the cost. Nor need they choose whether to have necessary hospital treatment on the basis of whether or not it is part of their insurance package. It is all covered under the Act, as long as it happens in the hospital and is medically necessary.

IV. Supplies and Equipment

It is not only the use of facilities and actual services that are covered. All the supplies and the equipment necessary for these hospital services—medical, surgical, or otherwise—are part of the public insurance scheme. This means everything from towels and toilet paper to bandages and oxygen masks, from hip replacements and heart monitors to clean sheets and diapers. There are no surprises at the end of the hospital stay in the form of a long, detailed list of every tissue and facecloth used. In fact, there is no record kept of such use by individuals.

V. Drugs and Other Preparations

Perhaps more surprisingly, drugs administered in the hospital are on the list. So are medications required for treatments considered as hospital services. So, too, are biological and other preparations, as long as they are part of hospital care. When a Canadian enters the hospital, no itemized list is prepared to include the whole range of drugs and other preparations required. The patient will receive the drugs the doctor orders, and the only difference between one drug and another for the patient is in terms of the consequences for their health. Whether the drug is aspirin or a sophisticated painkiller sold at a high market price makes no other difference to the patient.

VI. Health Care Providers

All these services, all the supplies, and all the equipment involve work by someone. The Act specifically names nursing services, a category which includes the work not only of the registered nurse but also that of every other kind of nurse from assistant to aide. (Private nurses have been rare in hospitals since medicare began, precisely because coverage was assured under the public scheme.) In addition to nursing, the Act explicitly includes those who interpret lab, x-ray or other diagnostic results. This means the full range of those who form the hospital diagnostics teams. Although these people in particular are singled out, the last item on the list of hospital services refers to everyone paid by the hospital. The Act recognizes that all the services provided by those working for the hospital are part of health care and thus should be considered as part of necessary services. Floors must be cleaned, food prepared and served, and records processed; all these are part of hospital health services and are therefore covered under the plan.

A Comparison of Canadian and U.S. Hospital Experiences

What does all this mean in practice? Judy Haiven, a Canadian journalist, was already working on a story intended to compare Canadian and American health care when her husband complained that he did not feel well. She rushed him to her local hospital emergency that Christmas holiday. In spite of a suspicion that Larry Haiven was simply suffering from holiday excess, the doctor kept him overnight for observation. But Larry's problem was much more than Christmas. He had a heart attack while in the hospital in Saskatoon, Saskatchewan.

The hospital responded with a full course of tests and treatments. Judy reports: "Monitoring in the cardiac care unit, followed by several days on the medical ward. Tests assigned: blood work, electrocardiogram, X ray, ultrasound, angiogram, exercise stress test, and others." Larry was prescribed medication to "ease the cardiac function and to 'thin' the blood."[3] When he was sent home, he was enrolled in a cardiac rehabilitation program and prescribed medication. For Larry, the entire process came without any bills. He paid nothing for this care, and neither he nor his family had the additional problem of finding out what his insurance would cover and how to pay for the rest. They had to worry only about his recovery.

As part of this recovery, the Haivens escaped the cold prairie winter to take a brief holiday under the sun. In California, Larry had more chest pains and was once again rushed to the hospital. This time, the clerk demanded payment before admission. Intervention by an American friend, his Canadian health care coverage, and permission from the clerk's boss finally got him into the hospital. Although this eventually proved not to be a second heart attack, Larry received virtually the same treatment in California as he had in Saskatchewan. The total bill from the U.S. hospital came to $12,590. "Everything had been itemized, right down to the sample-sized toothpaste ($5.25), the aspirin pill ($4.14), and the laxative ($17.04), which Larry didn't take."[4]

Judy had her story about the contrast between the Canadian and American systems. She went home to Saskatoon and asked the hospital what Larry's treatment had cost the system. The Canadian hospital estimated its costs at the equivalent of $US 3,500. For Larry, the only real difference between his experiences in Canada and in the United States concerned the unwelcome extra anxiety he felt south of the border. Would he get admitted to hospital promptly? Would there be hefty bills to pay? For the hospitals, it was another story. The same kind of care cost more than three times as much in the United States. Yet the care was virtually the same and equally comprehensive in both hospitals.

Doctors

The comprehensiveness principle applies to doctors as well. All medical practitioners who are entitled by law to practice medicine in Canada are covered by the Canada Health Act, and the Act includes insurance payments for all medically required services.

Most of what constitutes medical necessity is determined by physicians. In general, governments rely on physicians to decide what is required. Governments then pay for both the diagnosis and the treatment provided by the doctors. It does not follow from this principle that all medical services are covered. If the doctor determines that a service is simply a preference of a patient or an option that would be helpful but not necessary, then it would be outside the public insurance scheme. Such procedures would be paid for by the patient or the patient's private insurance coverage.

"Medically necessary" has no further specification in the Canada Health Act. There has been a great deal of resistance to providing any more detailed definition. Physicians have consistently argued that they alone have the knowledge to determine what any particular individual needs to maintain or regain health, or have a peaceful death. Any other agency involved in making the distinction would interfere with the autonomy that doctors not only value but require in order to provide appropriate care. Various citizens' groups have supported this position. Doctors are preferred to non-medical personnel as decision-makers, both because they have expert knowledge and because they can put the patient's needs first in a public system.

The National Forum on Health was equally convinced that a move to define medically necessary is not desirable. This government-appointed committee of prominent Canadians reported to the Prime Minister in early 1997 that:

Any list-based approach to defining medical necessity—with some things publicly funded and others not—will invariably be valid for only a short period of time due to the pace of technological change. Any list-based approach will carry with it the defects of its forebears, namely, the almost invariably flawed assumption that any service is either always useful or always useless (Hurley et al., 1996). The alternatives—attempting to define the circumstances under which a service is useful or not—have thus far been plagued with complexity while failing to solve the conceptual problems. One also has to question what role is left for professional judgment if insured services could be defined in such a precise, objective manner.[5]

Although the Act places no restrictions on the physician's right to decide, there are in practice some limits beyond those of the Hippocratic Oath. The fee schedule negotiated between doctors' associations and the provincial governments set out the kinds of services that will be paid for by the health insurance scheme. These fees cover an enormous range of diagnosis and treatment. They also primarily reflect what the doctors say is required, because governments have for the most part bowed to doctors' claims in terms of what is necessary. Governments have fought with doctors more about the fees paid for these doctor-defined services. Equally important, many of these negotiated services are quite broadly defined. Within these categories, it is the individual doctor who decides what is medically necessary.

The bills doctors submit are seldom scrutinized by the provincial governments. If the government does a random check, as some governments do, the purpose is mainly to determine whether the procedures did in fact take place. They are not about whether the procedures were appropriate or required. And doctors are seldom asked by the Colleges of Physicians and Surgeons to explain how they define medical necessity in a specific instance.

This situation contrasts sharply with that in the United States for doctors who operate outside public plans. Although doctors on both sides of the border have been heard to claim that public insurance means doctors lose their autonomy to bureaucratic decision-making, it is very difficult indeed to demonstrate that this has happened in Canada. Governments in Canada have not placed many restrictions on a doctor's right to decide what course of treatment is necessary, even though these same governments pay the bills. In the past, U.S. doctors billing Medicaid and Medicare have enjoyed similar freedoms.[6] But in the United States, insurance companies do regularly place restrictions on doctors' decisions. They do question doctors about whether certain procedures are required, and even in effect prevent them from acting on some decisions they make by refusing payment. Unlike the provincial governments in Canada, insurance companies in the U.S. often have doctors' diagnosis and prescriptions checked by others. And these others may be nurses or other providers who have less training than doctors or may be managers who have no medical training at all.

To sum up, public health insurance in Canada covers all aspects of care in the hospital and doctors' care outside the hospital. All the people, equipment, and supplies necessary for tests of any kind are covered. All the housekeeping services, food services, and transportation services are covered. So are all the drugs and equipment used, as well as the people who operate them.

Dentists

When the young Tommy Douglas was lying in bed recovering from surgery and making his vow about health care, he was thinking mainly in terms of doctors and hospitals. But an older Tommy made it clear that truly comprehensive care would have to extend beyond this. Part of Tommy's dream of including practitioners other than physicians and surgeons has been realized, although few participate on the same terms doctors do. This exclusion can, in large part, be explained by doctors' resistance to extending their privileges to others.

Dentists are the only other practitioners explicitly mentioned in the Canada Health Act. Like doctors, they are forbidden from extra billing for services covered by the public insurance plan. Perhaps more importantly, surgical dental services are included in public insurance if the procedures are most appropriately carried out in a hospital. In other words, dentists who do their work in hospital settings are part of comprehensive care, whether or not they are hospital employees. And this is clearly among the most expensive and necessary dental care.

Some dental services are also offered without charge through public health units across Canada. Traveling dental clinics have been initiated as part of provincial plans, with services provided to rural communities at little or no cost to the individual for some procedures.

Given its particular focus on health promotion, it is not surprising that Quebec introduced a comprehensive dental package for children. A whole range of services could be delivered by a dentist who then billed the government in the same way fee-for-service physicians do. In most provinces, welfare recipients are also provided with some essential dental care. These services too may be delivered when in the hospital or by self-employed dentists. In general, however, dentists in Canada are not part of the public insurance plan and do not negotiate a fee-for-service schedule with the government in return for guaranteed payment.

Because the public insurance plan does not cover most dentistry, private insurance firms are free to enter the field. Dental care is frequently part of the employee benefit packages negotiated by unions or offered to managers as part of their contracts. With dentistry, then, the Canadian situation is much like that more generally in the United States. The poor, most of those with good, secure jobs and their dependents are covered, while those with more precarious employment and their dependents are not. Although the terms for various sorts of dental coverage vary enormously, as a general rule those covered as part of their fringe benefit package at work have access to a broader range of services than those who receive dental care as part of their welfare benefits.

Other Practitioners

When the Canada Health Act was being debated, nurses in particular wanted to challenge the doctors' monopoly over the right to bill the government for services rendered. Although their personal financial interests certainly played a part, their argument was about more than gaining a share of tax dollars. It was about challenging the power of doctors and their exclusive focus on curative approaches to care. Optometrists shared the nurses' view that the reference to doctors should be replaced by "health professionals."[7]

Their position made sense to both the Minister of Health and the Standing Committee of Parliament that was examining the issue. Both were convinced by the evidence demonstrating that other practitioners could not only provide different kinds of care but also offer care that could be less expensive in the long term. Fears that responding to these demands would increase short-term costs and that doctors would strongly resist led to a compromise that nonetheless opened the door to more comprehensive care.

Medical practitioners retained their pride of place but the term "health care practitioner" was added. According to the Canada Health Act, the services of a whole range of other professionals "lawfully entitled under the law of the province to provide health services in the place of which the services are provided by that person" could become part of comprehensive care.[8] Moreover, the services could be offered anywhere, not just in hospitals.

For the same reasons that Monique Bégin had to compromise when as Health Minister she was introducing the Act, few provinces took full advantage of this addition. Doctors resisted and finance ministers worried that expenditures would soar if more practitioners could bill the government for care. The addition of the term "health care practitioners" nonetheless opened the door to alternative ways of delivering care, and especially to ways more in keeping with an emphasis on health rather than illness. The midwifery program in Ontario provides just one example of the potential inherent in the inclusion of other providers under the Canada Health Act. It is very much in keeping with Tommy Douglas's dream of transforming much more than the payment scheme.

Midwives

In the early part of this century, doctors viewed midwives with particular suspicion. These women not only took away important business. They also challenged the entire scientific basis of medicine with their traditional practices and their apprenticeship methods of learning. Equally important, midwives' services to women denied doctors vital access to families, access that could lead to lifelong care for the whole family in question. The doctors were successful in banning midwifery, and midwives virtually disappeared from the health care systems of the provinces.

The new midwifery movement that began to emerge in the 1960s was linked to the larger health promotion movement as well as to the women's movement. Midwives stood in direct opposition to much of orthodox medical practice. Instead of "delivering" babies, midwives "caught" them. This difference in language was intended to draw attention to their woman-centered practices and to the health promotion emphasis in their approach. Midwives worked in teams to provide continuous care and to offer women informed choices about where and how to have their babies.

Not surprisingly, these new midwives faced strong opposition from

71

a medical establishment that still saw them as a threat to medical practices and to the patient rosters of doctors. The midwives responded by countering the claims made by their medical opponents and by demonstrating the benefits of the midwifery approach. Among these benefits was a promise of lower-cost services resulting from a combination of less expensive procedures carried out in less expensive locations.

By the early 1990s, the midwives in the province of Ontario were successful. They are now registered to practice, with eligibility determined by a College of Midwives that is part of the province's system to regulate health professions. Their interests are protected by an association much like that of the doctors. And like the Ontario Medical Association, the Association of Ontario Midwives has negotiated payment terms with the provincial government.

Unlike the doctors with their fee-for-service system, however, midwives are paid annual salaries. For them, the fee-for-service approach promotes the wrong notion of care by dividing the body into parts to be fixed and care into treatment tasks to be performed on these parts. For midwives, appropriate care is continuous, integrated care for whole people, adjusted to meet their individual needs and preferences in the context of their social settings. On salary, midwives can better make mother, infant and family the sole focus of attention.

The midwives have negotiated a salary schedule that acknowledges their four intensive years of university-based education and their considerable responsibilities. In return for a full-time salary of $C57,000 to $C75,000 a year, a midwife works in a team of two or more members, attending at least forty pregnancies a year as the primary midwife and another forty as the back-up midwife. The births they attend can take place at home, in a stand-alone birthing center, or in a hospital. Midwives are able to admit mothers to hospital and to take full responsibility for them while they are there. They can also assist doctors if the mother chooses or if medical complications require additional medical intervention.

These alternative birthing sites have been negotiated for a number of reasons. First, they give mothers choices. Second, they allow midwives to advise mothers on the basis of diagnosed need. Third, they encourage midwives to seek the advice and assistance of doctors when this seems appropriate. And fourth, they enable the use of lower-cost sites when this is possible and chosen.

The licensing and funding of midwifery marks an important step towards a new model of care. Before its inclusion, only those women with significant financial resources could afford the expense, and risk, of midwifery services. Now midwives are on a solid economic foundation, and can offer their services without regard to the mother's financial circumstances. Each team of midwives begins to provide care soon after conception and continues after birth for several months until the mother is securely established with her child. This care includes a full range of services, from nutrition and exercise counseling, to clinical intervention to making arrangements for social support. Thus, choosing a midwife need not mean the absence of care directed by a doctor. Both midwife and doctor can be involved, especially if a delivery is complicated. The Canada Health Act allows this development of more integrated care in the case of births, and does so in a way that makes it accessible to women, without financial barriers.

Drugs

When Tommy Douglas first introduced public hospital insurance to Saskatchewan, penicillin had been in regular use for little more than a decade. Drug therapy and drug use were quite limited in health care and drug companies were, by today's standards, quite underdeveloped. Even by 1975, Canadians were spending only two-thirds as much on drugs of all kinds as they were on physicians. By 1996, however, Canadians spent just as much on drugs as they did on physicians.[9] During this same period, the amount spent per person grew from \$53.73 to \$361.95, an increase of well over 500 percent.[10]

A variety of factors, some more obvious than others, contributed to this shift in expenditures. As the number of drugs proliferated, more of them proved safe and effective at treating a wide range of health problems. At the same time, some of the drug therapies could be substituted for more traditional kinds of care. For example, patients could be sent home right after surgery, armed with drugs designed to prevent infections once prevented by nursing care. But it was also the case that these drugs were increasingly produced mainly by giant corporations with strong market positions, enabling them to raise prices and increase profits. In combination these developments resulted in drug expenditures that grew faster than any other category in the health budget. Public health insurance has expanded, in a limited fashion, to accommodate these developments. Current estimates indicate that public funds cover about 35 percent of all the money spent in Canada on prescription drugs.[11]

One source of government funding for drugs is hospital budgets. As we have seen, the Canada Health Act requires that drugs administered in hospitals be covered by public insurance. This is a very good way to ensure comprehensive care as long as drugs are administered within the hospital. As more and more drugs are prescribed through outpatient clinics, day-surgery facilities, and doctors' offices, however, fewer

Table 4.1
DRUG EXPENDITURES AND COVERAGE IN CANADA

Drug Expenditures	1975	1985	1996*
Drug expenditures as percentage of all health expenditure	10.2	10.7	14.4
Public share of drug expenditures	26	37.2	35.2
Private share of drug expenditures	74	62.8	64.8
Drug Insurance Coverage			**1995**
Percentage covered by public plans			44
Percentage covered by private plans			44
Percentage with no coverage			12

*Estimated by Health Canada

Sources: For drug expenditures: Health Canada, *National Health Expenditures in Canada 1975–1996: Fact Sheets* (Ottawa: Minister of Public Works and Government Services, 1997), tables 4 and 8. For drug coverage: National Forum on Health, *Canada Health Action: Building on the Legacy. Volume II, Synthesis Reports and Issues Papers,* "Directions for a Pharmaceutical Policy in Canada," p. 3.

and fewer drug expenditures fall under this part of the Canada Health Act.

Three provincial governments (British Columbia, Saskatchewan, and Manitoba) have moved to fill this growing gap in comprehensive care by introducing universal drug plans. A fourth (Quebec) is in the process of introducing a similar plan. In the jurisdictions with this approach, all residents are part of the drug payment scheme. Although the plans are universal, they do not provide free drugs to those who have prescriptions to fill. Unlike public hospital or medical insurance, public drug insurance comes with significant user fees. Indeed, in the judgment of the National Forum on Health, the deductibles are so high that relatively few residents actually obtain reimbursement.

User fees for public drug insurance take two forms that are familiar to those who enroll in private health insurance schemes. In the case of co-payments, patients pay either a fixed percentage of the bill or a fixed dollar amount on each bill. For co-insurance schemes, there is a maximum placed on the amount any individual or family must pay. Unlike much private insurance coverage, these plans do not have maximums on the total amount that can be billed, nor do they exclude people on the basis of prior health problems. In fact, several provinces now cover at least some of the costs of drugs in what are termed "catastrophic" situations. These are cases in which necessary drug treatment is both expensive and ongoing.

While only a few provinces have universal drug plans, most provide prescription drugs for the poor, the disabled, and the elderly. Some do so without any charge to the patient, while others require user fees. These targeted Canadian drug plans resemble the drug coverage provided in the United States through Medicare and Medicaid. Individuals must meet income, disability, or age criteria to be covered. Thus, those on welfare must pass a means test to become eligible. In the case of the elderly in Canada, only one province bases eligibility for drug payments on economic need. The others provide universal coverage, albeit usually with user charges.

With these limitations on universal coverage, there is plenty of room for private insurance schemes. Those people with such coverage usually acquire it through their place of employment. Approximately 44 percent of Canadians have private insurance, although not surprisingly those most likely to have coverage are those with full-time, stable employment in relatively well-paid jobs. A 1995 survey found that three-quarters of those with incomes over $60,000 had private insurance. Coverage dropped as income dropped, with only 7 percent of those earning less than $20,000 a year covered by private insurance. Just over one in ten Canadians had no coverage for drugs at all.[12]

The combination of more coverage and better health means that high-income households spend less on drugs, and these expenses make up a smaller share of their income than in low-income households.[13] As is the case in the United States, the poor pay more for their drugs and spend more of their income on drugs because there is no universal public plan.

Private schemes in both countries have complex arrays of deductibles and other kinds of user fees, as well as a wide variety of conditions related to eligible drugs. As a result, even those with private coverage end up spending money directly out of pocket to pay drug bills. One study estimated that about 65 percent of private expenditures on drugs in Canada are paid by private insurance schemes. This leaves individuals paying a significant proportion of the cost, even after investing in private insurance.[14]

Although the federal government has not taken steps to ensure universal drug coverage, it has intervened to regulate drug prices. Studies in the 1960s and 1970s demonstrated that Canadian drug prices were among the highest in the world. These prices were attributed to two main causes: lack of competition and foreign control of the drug market.[15]

In response to this research and to popular pressure, the federal government introduced changes to the Patent Act. These changes permitted licensed manufacturers to reproduce patented medicine once they had paid a royalty to the patent holder as determined by the Commissioner of Patents.

The strategy worked. A Canadian drug industry developed and some drug prices came down. The new "generic" drugs that provided lower-cost alternatives to "brand name" products helped provincial drug plans expand without exorbitant expenditure increases.[16] And they did so without significantly lowering the profits of the companies producing the "brand name" drugs.

Provinces, too, have developed strategies to control drug prices. In British Columbia, the government introduced a system called "reference-based pricing." All drugs that are used to respond to the same health problem, regardless of their chemical composition or the way they function, are assigned to the same reference class. If the research demonstrates these drugs are equally effective in treating the problem, then the province's universal drug plan pays only the cost of the lowest-cost effective drug. For example, one category for reference pricing covers drugs generally used to treat gastric disorders while another includes those usually prescribed for osteoarthritis treatment.

Many doctors and pharmacists claimed that the scheme would remove their ability to provide the most appropriate prescription for particular patients. In response to this concern, the plan allows physicians to request special authorization, authorization which allows full payment for a non-reference drug. Blanket exemptions for specific types of procedures or patients are also possible. This added flexibility provides more alternatives for both physicians and patients, based on demonstrated therapeutic concerns.[17]

Like compulsory licensing, reference-based pricing works at reducing drug costs. British Columbia's annual Pharmacare budget is approximately $350 million, and reference based pricing saved $21 million in the first ten months of operation alone. The plan "is also having a modest spin-off effect on [the] private health insurance market, reducing drug costs for private employee health plan carriers and consequently their employer plan sponsors."[18] At least as beneficial is the impact on physician prescribing patterns. There has been a significant shift to more cost-effective drugs. Because reference classes were based on the province's consultations with physicians and sub-specialty groups, as well as on the research literature, there is every reason to believe that this shift is consistent with good prescribing practices.

Not surprisingly, the manufacturers of brand name drugs have resisted this initiative. Their court challenge to the law failed, however. Meanwhile, some companies have lowered the prices of their more

77

expensive drugs in response to the competition from reference-based pricing.[19]

Joint purchasing by hospitals in some jurisdictions has also helped lower the cost of drugs for the government. Buying in bulk means not only that better prices can be sought by those hospitals but also that more pressure is put on prices in general. This kind of collective strategy is much more likely to develop in a public system where hospitals are not competing with each other for patients, as they are under for-profit conditions in the United States.

Government intervention, then, can have a positive impact on the distribution of drugs even without a universal plan. Combined with a universal plan, as is the case in British Columbia, government policies can have substantial impact both to control costs and to increase access without duly harming drug company profits. Indeed, cost-control strategies are crucial if universal plans are to be financially viable.

Quality Care

Maybe the fact that it is free to the individual makes people suspicious. Perhaps it's the notion that you get what you pay for, and if it's free, then it can't be worth much. It could be the idea that public health care means government issue, the same low standard for everyone. Whatever the reasons, critics have been quite skeptical about the quality of Canadian health services when compared to the quality of those in the mainly private American system.

There is, however, very little evidence to support the claim that Canadians get poor-quality care. In fact, there is very little evidence on the quality of care on either side of the border. Neither country has developed many effective ways of assessing the quality of services delivered. This is particularly surprising in the United States, given that it is assumed that a private system allows consumers to make choices on the basis of both quality and price. If you do not have the information necessary to evaluate the quality of services, it is difficult to make informed choices. Canada and the United States need better ways to evaluate how well their health services work at ensuring health and avoiding harm.

In spite of the paucity of quality information on quality, it is possible to make some comparisons. The limited evidence that is available indicates that Canadians get care that is at least as good as that south of the border.

Outcomes: Comparing Health

The most important measure of quality care must be health. As a host of research makes clear, health is determined by a range of factors. The most critical are food, shelter, jobs, and joy. Health services also have an impact though, so it is useful to look at the overall health of a population in assessing the quality of its health care services.

On such measures, Canada comes out ahead of the United States. Take babies, for example. More babies die in the United States. In 1994, 6 out of every 1,000 babies born in Canada died within the first year; this was the case for 8 out of every 1,000 American babies born that year.[20] In other words, out of every thousand babies born, almost two more died in infancy in the United States. Part of the explanation for this difference can be found in the number of very small babies born south of the border. Canadians babies are less likely than American babies to have low birth weights. Perhaps more significantly, while the proportion of Canadian babies with low birth rates declined between 1983 and 1993, the reverse was the case in the United States. In 1992, 5.5 percent of Canadian babies had birth weights under 2500 grams (5.5 lbs.) while this was the case for 7.1 percent of American babies.[21] Clearly factors such as nutrition and practices such as smoking are involved in low birth weights. But so are regular visits to doctors or midwives and obstetrical care. And these are without charge in Canada, suggesting that access to care may also be a factor. As for the mothers, they have a much better chance of surviving pregnancy and childbirth in Canada. Maternal mortality rates in the United States were almost double those in Canada in 1988, with 7 out of every 100,000 dying in Canada compared to 14 in the U.S.[22]

Canadians also live longer than their American counterparts. In 1995, for example, Canadian male babies could be expected to live for 75.3 years on average, while male babies in the United States could be expected to live 72.5 years. Women in both countries can be expected to outlive men on average, but Canadian women have the edge. They are likely to live to be 81.3 years, compared to 79.2 years for American women.[23] More importantly, Canadians have a better chance of living free of disability. By the late 1970s, Canadian women and men averaged 66 years of disability-free life. In the United States, both sexes averaged 60 years free from disability.[24]

Some of these differences may be related to differences in violent crimes and illicit drug use. There is more of both in the United States, although in 1984 U.S. drug-related deaths totaled just 30,000. Although 98,000 deaths in the U.S. were attributable to alcohol and 485,000 were attributable to tobacco, Canada's drinking and smoking rates were higher.[25] The conclusion to be drawn from this evidence is that some of the differences in life expectancy must be attributable to access to quality health care services.

The role of health services becomes more obvious when we focus on what the health system does best. There is a health gap between the two countries when considering only those illnesses that can be treated. Diseases of the circulatory system, including those of the heart, provide one example. In 1989, the years of potential life lost to Canadian women under age 65 from such diseases was 320 per 100,000, while for American females it was 538. Men in both countries lost more years to these diseases, but the differences between countries was still quite evident. The comparable data for males were 1020 per 100,000 in Canada and 1250 in the United States.[26]

Canadian babies, then, have a better chance of surviving, as do smokers, drinkers, and those with heart problems. Some of this must be related to the quality of, as well as access to, health services.

Hospital Care

Outcomes and quality are difficult to assess in terms of specific treatments and services. Canadians have more hospital beds per person, and stay longer in hospital than their U.S. counterparts. But do they get good care while they are there? Information on the quality of hospital care is scarce. There is an even greater shortage of data on the consequences of hospital care for patient health, especially if health is broadly defined.

The research that is available, however, indicates that Canadian hospitals offer high-quality services that stand up well to comparisons with the United States. In both countries, hospitals must be licensed by government agencies. So, although most hospitals are not government-run, they do need government approval to operate. To qualify for such a license, hospitals must meet certain minimum criteria. Independent agencies on both sides of the border offer accreditation that involves a regular assessment of services resulting in a certification of quality.[27] The accreditation process is much the same in both countries, suggesting that accredited hospitals offer very similar quality of care in Canada and the United States.

Comparisons of hospital staffing might imply that Americans receive more care, given that U.S. hospitals spend more on hospital care and given that the staff/patient ratios are higher than in Canada. Research on both kinds of resources does not however support the common sense notion.

According to one U.S. study, "Canadian patients have more frequent evaluation of their vital signs, more dressing changes, and more other services that are provided on a daily basis."[28] As for diagnostic services, Canadians received more of some while Americans received more of others. Canadians had more chest X rays and urine analysis; Americans had more blood tests and echocardiograms. Overall, however, U.S. hospitals did not provide more of these services.

The researchers suggest that one explanation for why more resources do not translate into more clinical care can be found in the number of American hospital employees who work in administration. In 1986, Canadian hospitals spent almost 30 percent less on administration, an issue discussed in chapter 6.[29]

Canadian hospitals may also be providing more skilled care that translates into more clinical services. Compared to those in the United States, Canadian hospitals employed 27 percent more registered nurses, and a smaller proportion of licensed practical nurses and aides.[30] The proportion of the more highly skilled nurses is therefore greater in

Canada—a distribution that may have important consequences for quality of care.

Clearly, Canadian hospitals provide considerable basic care to patients, in some cases more than U.S. hospitals. But what about the more complicated procedures, the ones that are likely to have more spectacular results and involve very highly skilled professionals? The answer is that Canadian hospitals rate quite well here, too. Canada does more heart and lung transplants per million population than does the United States, and more than Australia, Finland, France, Germany, Sweden, and the United Kingdom as well. Among all these countries, Canada came third in terms of the rate of kidney and liver transplants.[31] It is true that Canadian hospitals do significantly less heart surgery than do American ones, but this difference does not have much of an impact on survival rates, suggesting that more surgery does not necessarily mean better quality care.[32]

Surgery and medical care may be safer in Canada than in the United States. According to data collected by the Organization for Economic Cooperation and Development (OECD), in 1989 the incidence of abnormal reactions and misadventures during medical care in Canada was just half that of the U.S.[33] A comparison of surgery outcomes in a western Canadian province and an American eastern seaboard state indicated that, for nine out of ten procedures, the Canadians had better long-term survival rates. It was this study that President Bush referenced when he claimed that post-operative mortality was higher in Canada. However, much of the difference was explained in terms of short-term mortality rates for the special problems involved in getting people from remote parts of Manitoba to a major hospital for hip replacement operations. If the data for these patients are left out, the rest of Canadian surgery patients had a better chance of surviving for three years after surgery.[34]

Whatever the evidence on the quality of care, Canadians are quite satisfied with their hospitals. Just over 70 percent of them say they are very satisfied with hospital care, while this is the case for 57 percent of Americans.[35]

Doctor Care

How do you measure the quality of doctor care? One way is to look at preparation. In both Canada and the United States, doctors must graduate from a medical school accredited by the government, pass a national examination, and proceed through some post-graduate hospital training before they can legally practice medicine. Even then, a license must be obtained from a state or provincially approved administrative body. Specialists take additional training, with years varying in both countries according to specialty. Education, training, and licensing policies are so similar in the two countries that the credentials are virtually interchangeable.[36]

Another way to assess the quality of medical care is to look at how standards are set and enforced. Again, the countries are quite similar in terms of formal procedures. In Canada, "colleges" in each province determine the standards of practice and discipline members. Once the exclusive monopoly of physicians and surgeons who deliberated in secret, these colleges now have non-medical members representing a variety of constituencies, and for the most part the proceedings of disciplinary hearings are no longer secret. In the United States, the work of monitoring the quality of services is assigned to the physicians who sit on professional review organizations and medical societies that are supposed to discipline members. These processes are quite effective in ensuring that new doctors meet the minimum standards set by the medical profession. They are less effective in ensuring that all practicing doctors meet current standards. In neither country does the medical profession regularly monitor members to examine the ongoing quality of their services.

These monitoring and standard-setting authorities on both sides of the border have tended to be more reactive than proactive. They have focused more on responding to complaints than on actively encouraging appropriate care or on developing new standards. Partly in response to such criticisms, physicians in Canada have been involved in establishing various government-supported research centers intended to help physicians improve their decision-making practices. Organizations such as the Institute of Clinical Evaluative Sciences in Ontario, the Manitoba Centre for Health Policy and Evaluation and the Saskatchewan Health Services Utilization Review Commission collect and analyze data that provide a base for developing guidelines for practice. They also gather data that can be used to monitor overall consequences for the population of patterns in physician practices. Similar information is compiled for similar purposes by an array of agencies in the United States.

Unlike in the United States, however, this information has not also been used as the basis for utilization reviews of individual doctors that set treatment standards that doctors are required to follow. Governments and hospitals in Canada have been much less active than insurance companies and managed care organizations in the United States in imposing practice guidelines. This does mean that American doctors have less autonomy.[37] The issue of whether it means better quality of care is an open question.

It is difficult to assess the impact because most measurement focuses on cost rather than on care, on control rather than on quality. In Rhode Island, physicians rebelled against the imposition of Milliman and Robertson guidelines for precisely these reasons. According to these guidelines, developed by a Seattle-based consulting firm and used by health plans covering more than 50 million Americans, women who have a modified radical mastectomy must be sent home a day after surgery; those having a hysterectomy are to be discharged within two days. In one physician's view, these guidelines would mean that "a third of our hospital days would be deemed unnecessary by these criteria."[38] As a result, quality would decline.

When she testified before a House of Representatives Committee, Dr. Linda Peeno provided a vivid example of how imposed guidelines can reduce the quality of care. A former utilization reviewer for an HMO, she testified that "As a physician, I denied a man a necessary operation that would have saved his life. And this caused his death. No person and no group has held me accountable for this because what I did saved a company a half million dollars." The focus was on cutting costs, not quality care. "It became clear to me that I was expected to deny as much as possible—to keep a minimal denial rate and that if I didn't I would be shortly replaced."[39] For her, the guidelines too often meant denying care.

George Anders, the author of *Health Against Wealth,* does see problems in the old system that often encouraged over-treatment or poor treatment. However, he also sees problems with the impact of imposed guidelines on the quality of care. "I think their big problem is what happens when people get sick. What happens when people stop fitting the easy standardized formulas. It becomes a system where patients are looked at like little cells on a spreadsheet, and someone in a big tower makes medical decisions without really thinking about the impact on the individual human life."[40]

Dr. David Naylor, director of one of the Canadian research institutes involved in evaluating medical practices, suggests that the different "economic levers and motivations" in Canada mean that guidelines must be "less rigid, more flexible, and less confrontational" in this country. The influence on doctors would be less direct than in the United States.[41]

Policy makers in both countries are convinced guidelines can be important tools in developing better quality in health care. As yet there is no evidence, however, to demonstrate that imposed guidelines in the United States have significantly improved physician services or made them better than those available in Canada. In some cases, they appear to have reduced quality as part of the effort to reduce costs.

Although research on physician practices and their consequences for patients is limited, there are a number of studies comparing the way doctors treat heart disease in both countries; studies that offer some indication of the quality of care physicians provide. One of these studies found that coronary angiography and coronary artery bypass surgery tend to be used appropriately in both Canada and the United States.[42] A study that looked at approaches to acute myocardial infarction revealed that the more aggressive treatment in the United States did not improve reinfarction and mortality rates.[43] Another study of the same problem concluded that physicians in both countries responded in very similar ways to severe coronary heart disease, and differences were related to the treatment of less severe cases where Canadians were less likely to perform surgery. Canadians were also somewhat less likely to prescribe some medications, a possible explanation for why several studies indicate that somewhat fewer Americans suffer from activity-limiting angina after treatment.[44] In simple terms, Americans who have heart attacks are much more likely to be prescribed heavy duty drugs and to have surgery, but their chances of survival are no better as a result. Canadians are somewhat more likely to have chest pains later. What all this research suggests is that the quality of care heart patients receive from physicians does not differ significantly in the two systems.

As for the patients, Canadians feel they get quality care. Moreover, surveys suggest that Canadians are significantly more satisfied than Americans with the care they receive from physicians. Just over half of Americans indicate they are very satisfied with their medical care, compared to 73 percent of Canadians.[45]

Technology

It is clear that Canada has less of some high-tech medical equipment than does the United States. In 1991 for example, there were nearly twice as many machines per capita for scanning and imaging in the United States as there were in Canada.[46] What is less clear are the consequences of this technology for the quality of care. In these days of a blind faith in technology as the solution to all our problems it may seem heretical to suggest it, but more technology does not necessarily mean better care.

One reason to question the link between technology and quality is the lack of evidence on either effectiveness or appropriate use.[47] Some technologies have never been properly evaluated; others are often widely accepted while evaluation is in progress. Equally important, technologies may be oversupplied, and partly as a result used too frequently in cases where they are either not necessary or useless, or where another, older and cheaper method is at least as appropriate.[48] Perhaps most significantly, the technology may simply reveal problems for which nothing can be done.

Take the case of magnetic resonance imaging or, as it is usually known, the MRI. While in 1991 Canada had 1.2 of these very expensive machines for scanning the body for every million people, the

United States had 4.11.[49] This does mean that not everyone who wants an MRI in Canada can have one quickly.

At a conference in Canada recently, a woman claimed that her husband's case demonstrated the need for more MRIs. He had been diagnosed with malignant brain cancer on the basis of multiple tests and by several doctors. His doctors in Canada did not think his case warranted moving him to the front of the line for an MRI, given that there was no treatment for his condition. Desperate, her husband paid a thousand dollars for the procedure in the United States. The MRI confirmed the diagnosis of the Canadian doctors. The technology did not improve the quality of care he received, but its very presence suggested that something else could be done.

It is not only the presence of these technologies that may result in inappropriate use. It is also the money to be made. As an article in the *New England Journal of Medicine* points out, the proliferation of cardiac catheterization facilities in the United States may well be connected to the fact that a "high volume of procedures brought prestige and financial rewards to hospitals, physicians, and the vendors of medical equipment."[50] The more expensive the equipment, the greater the prestige associated with using it, even if the use is not warranted by existing evidence.

The presence of technologies tells us little about their distribution, either. Even when technologies may significantly improve health, their impact will be limited if those who need access are denied it because they must pay for the procedure. If you cannot use the technologies without paying, or if the insurance company refuses to cover the costs, then having the equipment does not make much difference to the health of those who cannot pay. For medically necessary procedures, this does not happen in Canada because everyone belongs to the same public insurance system.

Distribution may also be influenced by hours of operation and by location. If MRIs are available only from 9:00 A.M. to 4:00 P.M. four days a week, then access is much more limited than it is when the technology is in constant use. Similarly, the impact of technology is limited if there is an MRI on every corner in one city and virtually none in another. Provincial agencies in Canada are making efforts to ensure that this very expensive equipment is employed as many hours as possible. And a public system, as we shall see in a later chapter, makes it possible to organize both hours and location in ways that most efficiently use expensive equipment.

This is not to suggest that Canada has no high-tech medical equipment or procedures. Canadian hospitals have ranked first in the world in some very high-tech areas. The Grace Hospital in Ottawa is a world leader in cataract surgery, offering training in some of its techniques to doctors from the Mayo Clinic. Canada has pioneered is doing some kinds of transplants.

Rather, it is to argue that the quality of care cannot be assessed by listing how many machines or high-tech procedures there are in a country. Their presence tells us nothing about their effectiveness, their use or their distribution. Canada has a lot of high-tech equipment, although not as much as the United States. While it may well be the case that Canada could improve quality by purchasing more technology, there is no convincing evidence to demonstrate that quality in Canada suffers as a result of fewer machines.

Hospital Services Covered Under the Canada Health Act

a) accommodation and meals at the standard or public ward level and preferred accommodation if medically required

b) nursing services

c) laboratory, radiological, and other diagnostic procedures, together with the necessary interpretations

d) drugs, biologicals, and related preparations when administered in a hospital

e) use of the operating room, case room, and anesthetic facilities, including necessary equipment and supplies

f) medical and surgical equipment and supplies

g) use of radiotherapy facilities

h) use of physiotherapy facilities, and

i) services provided by persons who receive remuneration therefore from the hospital

5

Portability: You Can Take It with You

It may seem obvious to point out that people can fall ill or have an accident anywhere, but this obvious fact has quite important implications for health care coverage. Its recognition led those developing Canadian medicare to make portability a central principle of the system. Public health insurance coverage follows Canadians without a break from service to service, from job to job, and from province to province. It even provides some coverage outside the country.

Moving from Service to Service

Returning to Toronto after a couple of years away, Pat Armstrong realized she was overdue for her annual medical checkup. A phone call to a family practice clinic at Women's College Hospital resulted in an appointment with her family GP a week later. She arrived to be met by the registered nurse who works at the clinic. Here, she was weighed, her blood pressure was taken, and vaccines were administered. Central to this part of the appointment was a discussion of work and family, along with issues related to exercise, diet, birth control, and stress. Patients needing particular help in any of these areas can be referred to the Hospital's own wellness clinic, where the non-medical determinants of health are a central concern. Much of the charting was done by the RN, before she handed the file over to the physician.

The physician's work was focused more on the usual examinations, including a pap smear. This test Pat dropped off at the hospital lab on her way out. The physician noticed some spots on her face that might be, or could lead to, cancer, so an appointment was arranged with a dermatologist who works in private practice. Similarly, when the GP noticed some change in Pat's voice and considered other related symptoms, he suggested a visit to a throat specialist who works at another hospital. This too was arranged by the GP's office.

What to do about hot flashes was next on the agenda. The cartoon beside the patient's chair presents two sides to the debate about estrogen replacement therapy (ERT), clearly suggesting this is not necessarily the automatic course of action. Pat has already tried Evening Primrose Oil with only limited effect. The physician's response was to pull out a recent journal article summarizing the latest research on homeopathic approaches, and together they read the results. Pat and the GP agreed that more soy is appropriate. But given that Pat fits all of the categories indicating the likelihood of osteoporosis, the doctor also suggested that she read the literature on ERT. There is research indicating this therapy can help strengthen bones and, if Pat is willing to consider it after she reads the research, then the doctor will schedule a test to assess her bone density. At that point, a decision about the therapy could be made.

Pat's experience is not unusual in the Canadian health care system. She has ready access not only to the doctor's office but also to a whole range of related services. These services can be coordinated quite readily through the doctor's office, given that one card does all. The health card issued by the provincial system provides universal access to the full range of medically necessary services. While clinics in hospitals may be able to offer coordination more easily, the offices of doctors in solo practice can also make such arrangements. Because the insurance is provided through a single payer, the coverage is portable from doctor to doctor, from hospital to hospital, and from test to test.

Like managed care in the United States, an integrated package of services can be covered in a way that allows patients to use one insurer for a range of care. Also like managed care in the United States, the general practitioner provides the main access route to specialists. Unlike managed care, however, the services are not restricted to a particular group of providers. And unlike other private insurance plans, coverage is not limited to certain practitioners signed up with or acceptable to the company. Instead, the single-payer system makes it possible to carry coverage over the full range of services available under the plan. There is no limit on the number and kind of specialists the patient can see, as there is with managed care. The specialists do not have to be on the staff of the managed care organization, nor do they have to work in the same hospital or even the same area.[1] Virtually all doctors, as well as all hospitals, are "signed up" with the public health plan.

If Pat does not find the throat specialist satisfactory, or if she must wait several weeks to see this particular person, she can ask her doctor to refer her to another one. If the specialist at the other hospital orders tests, these can be done at either doctor's hospital. Portability in this sense means being able to take coverage wherever the physician and patient find the most useful and accessible services.

Moving across the Province or from Job to Job

Portability is not restricted to specific geographical areas. Increasingly, people commute long distances to work. Or they travel even longer distances at irregular intervals. Or they move for months, even years, to another location. Illness and injury do not necessarily occur near home, however, and often the need for health care cannot be planned. Like many of these people, Pat had moved out of Toronto for a couple of years. And like many of them, she needed health care while she was away. Her provincial health card from Ontario gave her immediate entry to the full range of services in Ottawa, her new home during these years.

Portability in this sense means moving throughout the provincial system. Because it is a public health system, people are rostered to the entire provincial system rather than to a single service organization or to a specific network of providers, as they usually are in managed care. This means that traveling for work need not mean moving away from access to paid care.

It also means that patients can travel to the services that are seen to be best for their needs. While she was living in Ottawa, Pat could still visit the specialist in Toronto who did her regularly required specialty tests, even though it was quite possible to find a new specialist in Ottawa.

This portability is particularly important for those Canadians who live in rural areas or small towns scattered throughout this enormous country. With portable insurance, they have access to medical services in major urban centers where a choice of specialists and a wider range of services are more likely to be found.

For those in isolated communities or needing transportation to large centers for complex procedures, the portability principle also means getting patients to services. Ontario, for example, has a particularly well-developed air ambulance service for this purpose. Indeed, it has become "a victim of its own success," scrambling to meet growing demands as it becomes better known and as the health care system evolves. In 1993, this service provided over 17,000 transfers. Almost all were patients, although there were also a few provider team and organ transfers, all carried out of course at no direct cost to the individuals involved. About 3,000 of the patients were in life-threatening situations, and another 4,800 were in stable condition but suffering from serious illness or injury requiring prompt attention. The rest lived in isolated areas of the province lacking health care professionals (and usually lacking roads as well).[2]

This portability of services within the province contrasts sharply with the American private system, which channels health care primarily through employment. This results in three major differences between the two systems.

First, Canadians are much less tied to their employers through health care coverage. Although Canadian employers do offer some health care benefits, these are extra to the medically necessary services provided under the public plan. To change employers, then, does not mean sacrificing the right to necessary care. Choosing a new employer is not related to coverage for basic health care services. Nor need it be related to the kinds of plan available or its conditions. Canadians therefore have more choice about moving from employer to employer as a result of their portable health care plan.

Second, work restructuring has little impact on health care in

Canada. In both countries, employment has become more contingent, that is, more precarious, temporary, and insecure. A growing number of jobs are part-time, short-term, or simply insecure. A majority of this contingent work is done by women; women who in their middle years are much more likely than men to need regular health care. Yet only a small proportion of such workers are likely to receive health insurance as part of their employment contracts.

Similarly, an increasing number of people in both countries are self-employed, partly as a result of companies restructuring to contract out services. As they are their own bosses, they are unlikely to have a health insurance package. Such coverage is available from private insurers, but the price is very high because individuals lack the power that companies have to negotiate lower premiums for group plans and because insurers face higher administrative costs enrolling individuals one at a time.

With portability, Canadians can be self-employed or part-time employees without losing their right to basic care. They may not have dental plans like many of their friends with secure jobs and they may not have an automatic right to a private room under the plan, but they will still be covered for a wide range of health care services. By contrast, being restructured into a part-time job or into self-employment in the United States often means losing health coverage. According to separate studies undertaken in 1987 and 1991, more than three-quarters of the uninsured were either employed adults or dependents of employed adults.[3]

Third, employment in Canada does not tie people to particular procedures or services. Increasingly in the United States, the employer or the insurance provider is pre-selected. By 1994, "more than half of all Americans whose employers provided health insurance coverage were enrolled in managed-care plans."[4] These plans can set the number and mix of specialists available, as well as the kinds of services eligible for coverage. Changing employers can mean changing health plans and thus changing providers.

With portability under the Canadian public plan, coverage is not linked to either employment or neighborhood, so Canadians have many more choices about services whatever their place of employment or indeed whether or not they are employed.

Moving from Province to Province

The division of powers and responsibilities in the Canadian federal system has the potential, as it does in the United States, to create problems for those moving temporarily or more permanently from jurisdiction to jurisdiction. The federal government in Canada is responsible for the health of the military, of inmates in federal penitentiaries, and for some First Nations (Aboriginal) people. For these groups, it is fairly simple for the federal government to ensure coverage when people move across the country. What is more complicated is the question of how to do this for the rest, given that each province continues to have its own health system. With provinces responsible for care, even with federal funding there may be considerable variations in terms of the fees and wages doctors and other providers negotiate. There may also be significant differences among provinces in the costs of particular services. For example, it may be cheaper to provide care in a small province such as Prince Edward Island where rents are low and the population relatively homogeneous than it is in a large city like Toronto where living expenses are high and the population very diverse.

The Canada Health Act, and the earlier legislation that led up to it, decided to address this problem in quite simple ways. Basically, the Act required that health care be portable from province to province.

If people move from province to province, they do not risk the loss of coverage. The Act stipulates that provinces must not require new residents to wait more than three months before becoming eligible for complete coverage under the health system in their new location. In the interim period, those who move remain eligible for coverage under the plan in place in the province they just left.

During the three months of possible waiting time, the new residents need not return to their old province in order to obtain services without charge. They can instead use services in their new place of residence. In this case, the bills will be paid by the province they just left.

The way this is done varies from province to province. For some jurisdictions, the process may be much like that in private insurance plans. The patient pays for the services and then bills the provincial health plan. In other jurisdictions, the bills are sent directly to the provincial agency by the service provider and the patient never sees the bill.

The protection for temporary residents in a province is quite similar. Coverage is paid for by their home province. To accommodate differences among provinces in terms of service costs, the Act stipulates that the amount paid is the approved rate in the province where the service is provided.[5] Provinces are permitted to negotiate among themselves to divide costs differently, leaving some flexibility in the system.

While portability is guaranteed, it is not without limit. The provinces were worried that too many people might shop around the country for services, ending up billing for health costs in the most expensive provinces. This would not only add to costs, it would also make planning more difficult. Responding to this concern, the Act allows provinces to require "prior consent of the public authority" that administers the insurance plan for "elective insured services."[6] Elective insured services are specifically defined to exclude services provided on an emergency basis or "in any other circumstance in which medical care is required without delay."[7] Even in the case of elective insured services, prior consent cannot be required if the services are not available on a "substantially similar basis" in the home province.[8]

In other words, if people need services because they become ill in another province or if they seek these services elsewhere because these services are not available in their home province, then no prior consent can be required. So, for example, if individuals in the small province of New Brunswick need heart transplant operations and if this complex procedure is not available in that province, then they do not need to ask the provincial agency before seeking the operation in a neighboring province. However, if the transplants are done in New Brunswick but the patients simply prefer treatment in Nova Scotia, then they would have to seek permission from the New Brunswick government to have the surgery performed outside the province but paid for by the province.

Portability in this sense means coverage in any jurisdiction, with few restrictions on use.

Moving around the World

Canadians travel a lot, on business and for pleasure. They are particularly likely to travel to the United States for either purpose. Indeed, many Canadians cross the border to shop for a day, and many stay much longer to escape the Canadian winters. Crossing the border, or leaving the continent, does not necessarily mean leaving the public insurance plan, however.

The Canada Health Act also provides for coverage outside Canada. Because costs and charges vary so much around the world, it is difficult to require provinces to pay whatever the going rate is in the country a Canadian happens to be in when they require health care. Instead, the Act stipulates that payment be based on the costs in the Canadian's home province for similar services. Comparable standards, the size of the hospital, and other relevant factors must be taken into account when establishing that amount, so some leeway is allowed to accommodate national differences or variations in service provision costs across provinces.

The extension of the public insurance plan outside Canada applies to temporary absences. Therefore, although provinces are required to provide coverage on the same terms to travelers outside the country as they are to those who travel within the country, there is a difference. Provinces can place time limits on how long people can be absent from the country and still be covered by the public health plan.

This has become an issue in Canada mainly because a significant number of retired Canadians spend several months each winter in the southern parts of the United States. Given the age of retirees, this group is particularly likely to need and use health care services while they are away. In response to this concern, some provinces have more narrowly defined temporary absences. With this qualification, Canadians still enjoy health care coverage when on brief trips outside the country.

Portability in this sense means Canadians can take a vacation without worrying very much about the financial consequences of having an accident while they are away.

Traveling for Care

The Canadians receiving care in the United States have been cited as evidence for the inadequacy of the Canadian system. The assumption is made that they must be seeking better quality care or avoiding waiting lines in Canada.

But most of those who receive care outside Canada do so because they develop their health problems while they are away. Only a small minority of Canadians who receive care in the United States do so by choice.[9] The majority are like Larry Haiven, the man who had his second encounter with a heart problem while vacationing in the United States. It is mainly the travelers who receive care in the United States, not people who travel to receive care there.

Some rare and specialized treatments are provided in the United States for Canadians, and paid for by the Canadian system. For a very limited number of procedures, it makes little sense to offer them in a country where the relatively small population means the numbers requiring such care are extremely small. Many American states do not provide these procedures either, and for precisely the same reasons.

With portability not only among provinces but outside the country as well, it is possible to ensure access without wasting resources on services that will be rarely used. This is particularly the case, as we shall see in the next chapter, when portability is combined with a publicly administered health insurance system.

6

Public Administration

Red tape, bureaucracy, endless forms and regulations, duplications and expenses. These are what often first come to mind with public administration. Yet the Canadian publicly administered health system has much less of all of these than you might think; and significantly less than the mainly private system to the south. The cost savings, as well as the reduction in administration and regulation, can be attributed mainly to the single-payer system.

Take the case of Jill Armstrong. At age eleven, she broke her leg while playing at school. She was rushed to the hospital by ambulance. Called away from their classrooms, her parents arrived to find her coming out of the x-ray room. Only after Jill was in traction did the nurse ask her parents to provide Jill's health card. There was one short set of questions to answer. When she was released three weeks later in a body cast, the hospital arranged for follow-up checks and for physiotherapy. To use any of these services, Jill only had to produce her card. There was no other paperwork, no phone calls, no agencies to coordinate. It was one simple package, made accessible by one single card.

Single Payer

The public administration principle in the Canada Health Act simply requires that the insurance plan "be administered and operated on a non-profit basis by a public authority."[1] This authority must be re-

Table 6.1
PUBLIC SHARE OF HEALTH SPENDING
CANADA, 1996

Health Expenditure Category	Public Share - Percentage
Public Health	100%
Physicians	99%
Hospitals	88%
Capital	72%
Other Institutions	68%
Other Expenditures	53%
Drugs	35%
Other Professions	14%

Source: Health Canada, "National Health Expenditures in Canada: 1975–1996: Fact Sheets" (Ottawa: Minister of Public Works and Government Services, 1997), Table 8.

sponsible to the government and have audited accounts. It is this agency that oversees the payment of health insurance. It is clearly not socialized medicine. The public authority administers payment. It does not operate the health care system.

What does the publicly administered plan pay for?

Public insurance pays for all of public health. What constitutes public health in Canada are government programs, operating at the provincial level and through semi-autonomous regional units. These agencies are involved in the traditional public health concerns such as health education, nutrition, school inspection, infection control, and inoculations. In recent years, they have also taken up such matters as breast screening, counseling for various cultural and racial groups, family violence, and mental health services for the elderly.

Unlike public health departments in the United States, those in Canada deliver few personal health services because these are provided mainly through medicare in hospitals and doctors' offices. Nevertheless, research comparing public health services in the province of Ontario with those in various U.S. jurisdictions found that Ontario spent significantly more on public health and provided more uniform standards of care than was the case in the United States. Ontario's higher costs were partly explained by the provision of considerable services in sparsely populated regions, while comparable areas in the United States had significantly less public health care.[2]

This is perhaps as close as Canada comes to socialized medicine, with all but one province employing their own dedicated staff and establishing priorities. Government involvement here has been reinforced by Canada's leadership in health promotion activities, especially after the 1974 report by Health Minister Lalonde that stressed future health improvements would come from prevention more than from cure.[3] Contrary to what might be expected of government agencies, however, public health units in Canada have taken the lead in community development and empowerment strategies that have frequently led to severe criticisms of government initiatives.[4]

Physicians come very close to public health in terms of how much of their money comes from the public insurance plan. Public money accounts for 99 percent of doctors' incomes. Included in this expenditure category are the fees for services paid to physicians and psychologists, as well as salaries or other payments made under plans such as workers' compensation. While the share of their income physicians receive from public coffers is almost the same as public health units, doctors have a radically different relationship to government. Doctors remain independent entrepreneurs, albeit ones who have their bills paid by the public insurance plans based on a negotiated fee. This is socialized payment perhaps, but it is certainly not socialized medicine.

The case of other professionals is quite different. Only 14 percent of their costs are paid by public insurance. Four out of five of these "other professionals" are dentists, almost all of whom work in private practice. A significant proportion of their income derives from private insurance plans, however. As for the rest of those in private practices, the chiropractors, optometrists, podiatrists, osteopaths, naturopaths, private duty nurses, and physiotherapists are less likely to be covered by any plan, although particular services provided by physiotherapists, podiatrists, and optometrists outside hospitals are covered by some public insurance schemes.

In terms of institutions, in 1996 the public insurance scheme paid for 88 percent of all hospital costs and over two-thirds of those in other institutions. The remaining 12 percent in hospital expenditures came from private insurance companies and individuals. These private expenditures in hospitals covered procedures and services not deemed medically necessary, such as private rooms, cosmetic surgery, and some forms of new reproductive technologies. There are also a very small number of private, for-profit hospitals in Canada which operate mainly in rehabilitation and extended care.[5]

The other institutions that have two-thirds of their costs covered include homes for the aged and nursing homes, as well as residential care for the physically or mentally handicapped and for those who are developmentally delayed or psychiatrically disabled. Also included are residential care facilities for those with drug or alcohol problems and for emotionally disturbed children. The proportion paid for from the public funds varies with the kinds of clients, although a significant amount of the costs in all of them is paid for from taxes. More of these facilities are government operated than is the case with hospitals. Almost a quarter of the beds in residential care facilities are in municipal or provincially run institutions. But it is also the case that a much higher proportion of these institutions are privately operated for profit, accounting for a third of all beds.[6]

The public plan also pays for nearly three-quarters of the capital costs for construction, equipment, and machinery, with much of the re-

---

Table 6.2

**OWNERSHIP OF RESIDENTIAL CARE FACILITIES
CANADA, 1993**

Ownership	Share of beds – Percentage
Voluntary lay body, nonprofit	37 %
For-profit	33 %
Government	23 %
Religious, nonprofit	7 %

Source: Statistics Canada, *List of Residential Care Facilities 1993*. Cat. No. 83–240 (Ottawa: Minister of Industry, Science and Technology, 1994), Table 1. Includes care for the aged, physically handicapped, developmentally delayed, and psychiatrically disabled.

---

maining money coming from charitable donations. As for the rest of health expenditures, the public plan covers just over half. The proportion of cost covered within this category varies enormously not only from service to service but also from individual to individual and from province to province. So, for example, the plan in the province of Manitoba pays for a wide range of home care services, covering virtually all of the costs. In Ontario, people on social assistance may have the full cost of their eyeglasses covered while those with fulltime employment may have their glasses paid for by a private insurance plan.

Finally, public insurance covers less than half of all prescription drug costs. As we have already seen, most of these expenditures are made through hospitals or for individuals who are elderly or on welfare programs. The rest of the money comes from either private insurance or from the pockets of individuals.

In terms of public money then, the majority goes to doctors and hospitals although other expenditures are also part of the package. Private money is spent mainly on drugs and other professionals.

Table 6.3

PUBLIC AND PRIVATE SECTOR HEALTH EXPENDITURES BY CATEGORY CANADA, 1996

Category	Distribution of Public Spending	Distribution of Private Spending
Hospitals	43 %	14 %
Physicians	21 %	1 %
Other Institutions	10 %	11 %
Other Expenditures	8 %	17 %
Drugs	7 %	31 %
Public Health	7 %	0 %
Capital	3 %	2 %
Other Professionals	2 %	25 %

Source: Health Canada, "National Health Expenditures in Canada 1975–1996: Fact Sheets." (Ottawa: Minister of Public Works and Government Services, 1997), Tables 6 and 7. Columns may not add to 100 percent due to rounding.

How Much Does It Cost?

There are various ways to answer the question of public health care costs. One way is to look at the cost of health care goods and services exchanged as a percentage of all goods and services exchanged, or of what is known as the Gross Domestic Product (GDP). In 1995, Canada spent 10 percent of GDP on health, compared to 14 percent in the United States.[7] By this calculation, Canada ranks third among industrialized countries in terms of the share of the formal economy going to health.

If, instead of GDP share, we look at expenditures per person, Canada ranks fifth among Western countries, when these expenses are adjusted to reflect purchasing power. In 1995, Canada spent $2,049 per capita, or about 55 percent of what Americans spent per person.

But these figures give a very false picture of what the Canadian public system costs. All these measures refer to total spending and thus include both private and public expenditures. A much better way to look at the Canadian system is to focus on public costs and the share paid for from the public purse. In 1995, Canada's governments spent just under 7 percent of the GDP on health, a figure that is not very different from the 6.6 percent that comes from tax dollars in the United States. Indeed,

Table 6.4
HEALTH EXPENDITURES IN CANADA AND THE UNITED STATES
1995

Expenditure Rates	Canada	United States
Percentage of Gross Domestic Product	9.6	14.2
Public spending on health as percentage of GDP	6.9	6.6
Percentage of tax dollars spent on health	14.5*	16.4**
Spending per capita	$2,049	$3,701

Source: OECD, "Health Data 97," (OECD, Paris, 1997), Health I table.

* 1994. ** 1993

governments in the United States spend more of their revenue on health than is the case in Canada, almost 2 percentage points more. Although the proportion of public money spent in Canada and the United States is very similar, Canadians get much more for their health dollar and many more Canadians receive care from these public expenditures. As we have seen, this public money covers every Canadian for a wide range of services. In contrast, less than 30 percent of Americans are covered by government Medicare (13 percent), Medicaid (12 percent), and military (4 percent) care plans combined.[8] Yet the proportion of tax dollars spent is higher.

Another way to look at costs is to look at what individuals pay. For services covered by public insurance, most Canadians pay nothing. Unlike Medicare and Medicaid in the United States, there are no deductibles or user fees, no limits related to contributions or nature of the plan, no restrictions on which of the insured services can be used, and no means tests. For most there are no premiums to pay for basic care, only taxes.

Such an answer leads to a question about taxes. Have taxes increased enormously to pay for health care? This is a difficult question to answer, given that a special health tax was not introduced along with medicare and no clear connection can be drawn between tax rates and health expenditures. It is also difficult to compare taxes within Canada, let alone across countries or with the United States.

We do know that Canadian taxes are not particularly high. According to the Department of Foreign Affairs and International Trade, Canada's taxes are below the average for industrialized countries. And they are not significantly out of line with the United States. In terms of individual income tax rates, Canada's range from 25 to 54 percent, while those in the U.S. start at 15 percent and reach up as high as 52 percent, when all levels of government are taken into account. Corporate rates are even more similar in the two countries.[9] However, when it comes to payroll taxes, Canada has the lowest rate of the seven largest industrial countries, with a rate almost 2 percentage points below the United States.[10] Canada also has a sales tax that ranges from 7 to 18 percent. In the United States, there are federal excise taxes and state taxes that go as high as 8 percent. Here, then, Canadian rates are higher in some areas although this cannot be linked directly to health care costs.

Corporate, individual, and sales taxes tell most of the story of payment in Canada but not in the United States. For necessary care, Canadians cannot buy insurance coverage and therefore have virtually no costs. In contrast, most Americans must pay individually, through workplace coverage or both for necessary care. It is mainly coverage for necessary health care that explains why Canadian employers pay significantly less for benefits. A 1994 survey found that "As a percentage of gross annual payroll, Canadian employers in the private sector pay 34.9% for employee benefits, less than United States employers who pay 40.2%."[11] By 1990, American "corporations will spend more for health benefits than they retained in profits," although this was not the case in Canada.[12]

Once all the costs paid by individuals in the United States are included, Canadians individually pay significantly less than Americans for health care. Canadian taxes are somewhat higher if we ignore the costs of benefit packages and payroll taxes, but a progressive tax system helps ensure that the poor and sick do not pay a much greater share of their incomes on health than do the wealthy and the healthy, as is the case in the United States.[13]

Table 6.5
TAXES IN CANADA AND THE UNITED STATES
1996

	Canada	United States
Corporate taxes	15.6 – 46.1%	15 – 46.25%
Payroll taxes	5.9%	8.7%
Employee benefits	34.9%	40.2%
Individual income	25.2 – 54.2%	15 – 51.6%

Sources: Canada, Department of Foreign Affairs and International Trade, "Overview of Taxation in Canada, the United States and Mexico." World Wide Web, p. 1 of 25 (August 8, 1997); *CCPA Monitor,* "Canada's 'Payroll Taxes' Lowest Among all G7 Nations," (February 1997), p. 24; and KPMG Canada, "Benefit Cost Survey," World Wide Web, (August 8, 1997).

Table 6.6
FEES PAID TO DOCTORS

	Alberta (AHCIP)	U.S. Medicare Plan	U.S. Private Insurance or Out-of-pocket payers
EKG (heart tracing)	$23.75	$57.75	$71.25
Colonoscopy (bowel exam)	$99.87	$315.00	$590.00
Echocardiogram (heart exam)	$194.84	$723.00	$885.00
Cataract removal with lens implant	$503.13	$856.00 plus $230.00	$2600.00*

Source: Consumers Association of Canada (Alberta), *Consumer Watch*, (Fall 1996), p. 1

*Patient also pays $1900.00 facility fee and $750.00 anesthetic fee for 7–12 minute surgery.

Yet another way to answer the cost question is to compare what is paid for individual services. The above table, prepared by the Consumers Association in the province of Alberta demonstrates the significant differences in fees paid to doctors by various plans.

While it is the case that doctors receive significantly less from the Alberta plan, the doctors also pay out significantly less in administrative costs and malpractice fees. They also have guaranteed payment from the government and thus have no unpaid bills. They also spend less time doing administrative work and therefore can see more patients. The result is less-expensive care for the patient, as well as for the government and insurance companies.

Where Does the Money Come From?

The short answer to the question about sources of money for public health care is taxes. The overwhelming majority is raised through general revenues. A couple of provinces designate part of the taxes employers pay as a health contribution, and a couple charge fixed premiums to those who can pay. But these taxes are mainly about politics rather than expenditures on health or rights to health. The provinces that have health premiums or health taxes mainly keep them to remind people that the government is paying for health care.

The money designated as health money is not kept in a separate pot for health care; it is simply folded into the overall revenue of the province. These premiums and taxes bear virtually no relationship to whether or not people receive health care, given that all people must be covered. Nor do they bear any relationship to the kind or amount of care people can access, because care must be comprehensive for everyone. In any case, the amounts collected through these specified sources make up only a small portion of what is paid for health care from the public purse. As a result, the majority of provinces do not bother with either health taxes on employers or individual premiums.

All levels of government contribute to health expenditures but most of it comes from the provincial governments. As we have seen, health care is a provincial responsibility and the national program began when the federal government promised to pay half of specified expenditures as long as provinces met the five principles. The federal government provided half the cash for whatever was spent in the appropriate categories and in appropriate ways. The provinces simply had to submit their bills, much as physicians do today.

In some ways, this kind of funding was like writing a blank check although provinces still had to put up their 50 percent share. Worried about the open-ended nature of the funding process, about the stress on acute care, and about the administrative costs involved in checking the bills, the federal government introduced a new formula in 1977.

This new formula had several parts. First, there was a per capita payment, based on past practices and adjusted regularly to take the growth of the economy into account. Second, the federal government transferred to the provinces some of the national government's right to tax. This transfer of "tax points" allowed provincial governments to raise more revenue. This led directly to a third part, equalization payments to compensate for provincial differences in ability to tax. The fourth part was an additional, indexed, per capita payment to help pay for residential and home care, as well as for the ambulatory care that began growing significantly during this period. The arrangement was designed to encourage innovation, while discouraging acute care use.

In effect, the formula put a limit on federal spending. At the same time, however, it allowed for both new developments and for population growth. The federal government no longer checked the bills, reducing its administrative cost. During the following years, the federal government kept gradually lowering the overall amount allocated in cash while increasing the proportion defined as tax point transfers. The money was still designated for health, however.

This changed with the introduction of the Canada Health and Social Transfer in 1996. The legislation lumped together payments for health, post-secondary education, and social assistance, in the process further reducing the federal involvement in health expenditures. In effect, the provinces now receive a lump sum payment along with their tax points.

Table 6.7
SOURCES OF HEALTH SPENDING
CANADA AND THE UNITED STATES,
1993

	Canada	United States
Public	73 %	43 %
Federal★	25 %	31 %
Provincial/States	46 %	12 %
Municipal/Workers' Compensation	2 %	
Private	27 %	57 %

Sources: Health Canada, *National Health Expenditures in Canada, 1975–1994: Summary Report* (Ottawa: Supply and Services Canada, 1996), Table 2C; and Stephen M. Ayres, *Health Care in the United States* (Chicago: American Library Association, 1996), Figure 1–3.

★For Canada, federal includes direct expenditures and transfers to provinces.

The funding changes have meant that now provinces provide most of the money for care, albeit with taxes they collect in what were formerly federal jurisdictions and with money from the Canada Health and Social Transfer. In 1996, federal government direct expenditures on health for groups such as Aboriginals, the armed forces, and veterans, as well as for research, amounted to only 5 percent of all public spending. The national government contributed much more in tax transfers and cash to the provinces. The exact calculations are impossible to make for 1996 because the funds are now amalgamated. In 1993 such transfers made up 22 percent of all health spending. Nominally, then, the provinces account for 92 percent of public spending. Municipalities and workers' compensation pay for the rest.[14]

Here, the contrast with the United States is quite striking. In the United States, the federal government contributes much more than the states. At the same time, private sector spending in the United States makes up well over half of all health expenditures, compared to less than a third in Canada.[15]

Table 6.8
**FINANCING AND DELIVERY SERVICE
CANADA, 1994**

Service Type	Financing	Delivery
Hospital services	100 percent public for medically necessary services (no user charges permitted); private payment for upgraded accommodation or non–medically necessary services provided in hospitals	Mixed public/private. Varies across provinces. Government generally exerts a strong regulatory presence.
Physician services	100 percent public for medically necessary services (no extra-billing permitted); private payment for non–medically necessary services	Private—physicians are independent and self-regulating; some models of primary care delivery (e.g., CLSCs or community clinics in Quebec) are more akin to government agencies

Table 6.8 (*continued*)
FINANCING AND DELIVERY SERVICE
CANADA, 1994

Service Type	Financing	Delivery
Services provided in private clinics	Privately funded for services not defined as medically necessary. Some clinics charge a facility fee to patients for medically necessary services over and above the funding provided by the provincial health insurance plan.	Privately owned and operated—limited regulation
Dental and optometry care	Mostly private (insurance or out of pocket); some provincial plans provide coverage for children and seniors.	Private and self-regulating—e.g., dentists and optometrists
Prescription drugs	Mixed public/private; provincial plans pay for approximately 40 percent of all prescription drugs dispensed outside hospitals. Coverage is typically limited to seniors and welfare recipients. Drugs dispensed in hospitals are covered in hospital budgets. Balance is funded by a combination of private insurance plans and out of pocket payments.	Private—delivery includes prescription by physician and dispensing by pharmacist or hospital.
Non-prescription drugs	Mostly private (out of pocket)	Private—over-the-counter
Services of other professionals	Mostly private (insurance or out of pocket)	Private (e.g., psychologists, physiotherapists, chiropractors, midwives, private duty nurses).

Table 6.8 (*continued*)
FINANCING AND DELIVERY SERVICE
CANADA, 1994

Service Type	Financing	Delivery
Alternative medicines	Mostly private—some limited coverage provided by provincial plans; remainder is paid for through private insurance plans and/or out of pocket.	Private—e.g., naturopaths, homeopaths, practitioners of oriental medicine, traditional Aboriginal healers.
Long-term care (residential)	Mixed public/private; public portion covers insured health care services; private portion covers room and board.	Mixed public/private
Home care	Partial public coverage provided in most jurisdictions; informal caregivers play an important role.	Mixed public/private
Ambulance services	Partial public coverage in some provinces; special programs for residents of remote areas.	Mostly private operators
Public health programs	Public	Public
Services to Aboriginal peoples	Public	Mixed public/private (federal government employees deliver some services directly).

Source: Canada, National Forum on Health. "The Public and Private Financing of Canada's Health System" (Ottawa: National Forum on Health, September 1995), pp. 6–7. Note that the figures given here differ slightly from those in Table 6.1 because they represent different years.

Why Canadian Care Costs Less

The simple answer to the question about why Canadian health care costs less is that so much of it is publicly financed. Before medicare, there were no significant differences in what Canadians and Americans spent on health care services. Since the introduction of medicare in Canada, the differences in expenditures have steadily and significantly increased. What the Canada Health Act calls "public administration" has kept Canadian health care spending under control while providing quality care to the entire population.[16] There are several reasons why public administration makes for cheaper care.

Administrative Costs

One of the most important areas for cost savings is in administration itself. Recall that when Larry Haiven was released from a U.S. hospital after his heart attack scare, he received an itemized bill, detailed down to the sample tube of toothpaste, the aspirin pill, and the laxative he didn't take. In Canada, Larry did not receive a bill at all after his first hospital stay with a real heart attack. The Canadian hospital had no reason to collect the kind of details he was later to receive from the U.S. hospital. It would have been wasteful to go to the trouble of allocating the cost of insignificant items like toothpaste tubes to individual patients. Indeed, it would have been wasteful to allocate the cost of medications or surgical supplies to individual patients. Instead, the hospital simply purchases the supplies it needs and in turn provides them to the patients who need them.

Hospitals in Canada save on administrative costs not only because they do not have to keep detailed accounts for each patient, but also because they do not have to send each of them, or their private insurer, a bill. Moreover, Canadian hospitals do not have to send out these bills according to the different criteria and forms used by different insurers, do not have to worry about whether they can collect, and do not have to calculate how many "charity" cases they can afford to take on.

All this contrasts sharply with the situation in the United States, where, according to one study, hospitals "must keep more extensive

113

records in order to facilitate billing to the state and federal governments, insurance companies and patients, and in anticipation of malpractice suits." Comparing hospitals in California and Ontario, this
study estimated that "roughly half" the difference in hospital costs
could be explained by higher administrative expenditures south of the
border.[17]

Americans David Himmelstein, James Lewontin, and Steffie Woolhandler have examined how these administrative cost differences translate into personnel cost differences.[18] Their analysis demonstrates that
the significant differences in the amounts spent on administrative staff
in the Canadian and U.S. health care systems occurred only after the
Canadian system became fully publicly administered in 1971. As
shown in table 6.9, the staff totals were comparable in the two countries that year. When controlled for population and translated into full-
time equivalents, the United States had just over 7 percent more
administrative staff. By 1986, the United States had almost 42 percent
more. About a quarter of U.S. health care workers do "mostly paperwork," and this share continues to rise. "If the United States duplicated
Canada's 1986 staffing patterns, the country's hospital and outpatient
facilities would require 1,407,000 fewer clerks and managers."[19]

Two other points made in the Himmelstein et al study should be
mentioned here. First, their data exclude the quarter million Americans
who work for health insurance companies, and the tens of thousands
more who work on health benefits in the personnel departments of
large employers and at the corporate headquarters of hospital and nursing home chains. Second, in 1986 the U.S. health care system employed slightly *fewer* non-administrative staff to do the actual work of
looking after patients than did the Canadian system, if the figures are
calculated in relation to population size. In particular, the Canadian
system employed a lot more registered nurses, to pay skilled attention
to patients rather than to accounts.

As well, Canadian doctors do not have to keep different kinds of
records in their offices for different payers. Nor do they have to send
separate bills to individual patients. Like the hospitals, doctors get paid
for their medically necessary services by a public agency, and thus have

Table 6.9

ADMINISTRATIVE STAFF IN HEALTH CARE
CANADA AND THE UNITED STATES, 1971 AND 1986
(FULL-TIME EQUIVALENTS PER MILLION POPULATION)

	1971		1986	
	Canada	United States	Canada	United States
Managers & related	569	974	1425	2634
Admin. support, except financial	3082	3123	3778	4593
Admin. support, financial	430	280	604	999
TOTALS	4081	4377	5807	8226

Source: David U. Himmelstein, James P. Lewontin and Steffie Woolhandler, "Who Administers? Who Cares? Medical Administrative and Clinical Employment in the United States and Canada," *American Journal of Public Health* 86:2 (February 1996), table 2.

only that single agency to deal with for payment. No administrative effort is wasted in doctors' offices chasing after patients or their insurance companies for payment. No prior approval is required when ordering or providing specific health care services. No time is wasted discussing with patients the potential costs of treatments and whether they can be met. Doctors can spend all their time with patients on issues of care, and can spend much less money in their offices on administrative support.[20]

As one Canadian doctor who tried practicing in the United States explained, "I wasn't making any more money [in the United States]. My overhead was so much higher." He returned to Saskatchewan after two years in Idaho, not only because he made less but also because, south of the border, "People did not come until they were very ill," in order to avoid the expense of care. The result was more expensive, complicated, and drastic care. For example, this doctor could recall only one occasion during his 11 years of practicing in Saskatchewan when a leg had to be amputated because of complications with diabetes. It happened four times during his brief stay in Idaho.[21]

Administration also costs less in Canada because no effort is required to separate the eligible from the ineligible. No time is taken up with means tests to determine who qualifies for Medicaid, or with filling out forms to make sure applicants are old enough for Medicare. No time is spent ensuring that insurance coverage is up to date, that the right hospital is being used for a specific insurance plan, or that the required service is covered by that plan. Because all Canadians, and most health care services, are included in the public health insurance scheme, these kinds of scrutiny to assess eligibility are largely unnecessary.

By combining public administration with care that is universal, accessible, comprehensive, and portable, the Canadian medicare system can simplify its administrative processes enormously. It has little red tape, and fewer forms. It also has relatively few regulations. In a recent editorial in *The New England Journal of Medicine,* Jerome Kassirer reports that "at last count some 1,000 bills to control health plan practices have been introduced in 39 states and approximately 100 have been introduced in Congress" to protect the public, to require benefits, and to address the issue of doctors' authority under new managed care plans in the United States.[22] Proposed and enacted regulations include detailed directives on:

access to specialists, coverage of emergency care, length of maternity hospital stays, "gag rules" imposed on physicians by HMOs, prompt and fair appeals procedures for alleged wrongful denials of care, the availability of information about HMO plans, and travel and waiting time standards for care.[23]

Such regulations are simply not needed in the system organized under the short but clear Canada Health Act. It is private, targeted insurance that generates regulations and red tape, forms and restrictions, not public insurance.

In the Canadian system, hospitals and doctors are not alone in enjoying light administrative loads. Patients also have much less paperwork to fill out than do their U.S. neighbors. Canadians sign up but once for medicare, receiving one identification card good for the entire range of services. This card is all they have to produce when they enter the hospital, visit the doctor, or use any of the other services available under their provincial program. There are no bills to juggle at the end of the month, no calculations to make about which insurance company to choose or to charge. It is not possible to produce numbers on the amount of time individuals save under the Canadian system. Data of this sort cannot be accurately measured. Suffice it to say that a publicly administered and universal system means less paperwork, as well as less anxiety about how to pay the bills, than does a private, targeted insurance system.

A Nonprofit Basis

Another reason the Canadian health care system can keep costs down is that the delivery of the care is provided primarily on a nonprofit basis. As we have seen, the Canada Health Act requires only that the health care insurance plan of each province be administered and operated on a nonprofit basis by a public authority responsible to the province and subject to financial audit by the province's own auditor.[24] Although for medically necessary services "private insurance is implicitly or explicitly forbidden and there is no opting-out of paying taxes for the public system," the Act does not prohibit for-profit firms from *delivering* these services.[25]

It is possible, then, for the public authorities to purchase the delivery of care from for-profit agencies. This is most commonly done in the area of residential services, such as long-term care, substance abuse centers, and facilities for the developmentally disabled. Most health care, however, is provided by nonprofit organizations from public funds. With one payer, it is possible to give preference to nonprofit delivery and, further, to establish nonprofit status as a prerequisite for public payment. It is this combination of public administration and nonprofit care that helps keep costs under control and lower than those in the United States.

For-profit care in a primarily private funding system, or even in a public funding system, can increase costs in a number of ways. First, and most obviously, a share of the expenditures goes for profits, and what goes to profit does not go to care. Companies in the United States involved in selling health insurance and, increasingly, the delivery of health care services, are enjoying what Jeanne Kassler calls "stratospheric profits."[26] In 1996, for example, Merck recorded a net profit worldwide of $US 3.9 billion, or $79,000 for each of its 49,000 employees. And it was not the only drug manufacturer with high profits. Roche showed a profit of $64,500 per employee that year, while Glaxo Wellcome trailed at a mere $57,000.[27]

And the high profits were not by any means limited to the pharmaceutical sector. "Medical loss ratios" is the curious term used by health maintenance organizations and insurance companies to refer to the share of their revenue they have to pay out for actual health care. According to one study, for eight large HMOs this ratio fell from 89 percent in 1987 to 78 percent in 1994.[28] Not all of the remaining 22 percent shows up as profit. There are some necessary administrative costs. And then there are the million-dollar-plus salary, bonus, and stock option packages for their senior executives. The compensation of the chief executive officers at 70 of the largest U.S. health corporations averaged $1.5 million in 1995.[29] Finally, there is profit: $US 1.13 billion of it for the six largest California HMOs in 1994 alone, giving them accumulated cash reserves of $5.6 billion.[30]

For the senior executives of hospitals, HMOs, and the like, the money really starts to roll in when a corporate takeover occurs. To take an extreme recent example:

Leonard Abramson, CEO of U.S. Healthcare, will get more than $967 million in cash and stock, plus a $25 million corporate jet and a $10 million consulting contract, from the firm's purchase by Aetna. Two of U.S. Healthcare's co-presidents will receive an extra $11.62 million in cash and stock for joining Aetna.[31]

By early 1997, Aetna had 4.1 million "members" or subscribers making it the third-largest publicly traded HMO in the United States.[32] But the action is not limited to giant corporations. When the Physician Corporation of America (PCA) bought Better Health Plan of Coral Springs, Florida, with its 48,000 members for $8.2 million in 1992, it also paid the three former owners $5 million in consulting fees and "non-compete agreements."[33]

Relative to the average pay that goes to workers, the remuneration of senior executives is generally much higher in the United States than in other industrialized countries, including Canada.[34] This difference is particularly evident in health care. The provincial health insurance plans in Canada are run by civil servants at civil servant–level salaries. Only a handful of hospital CEOs earn as much as $US 200,000. And while there are fringe benefits that must appear very generous to a hospital laundry worker, there are no fat bonuses or stock options available to senior hospital executives.

In addition to profits themselves and the funds channeled to senior executives, the search for profit has other disadvantages in health care. It leads to waste and to inappropriate care. Profits are derived both from reducing costs and from increasing sales. It is consequently in the interest of for-profit firms to sell as much expensive care as possible, rather than to focus on providing appropriate services as determined on the basis of health care needs. In *Health Care in the United States: The Facts and the Choices,* Stephen Ayres describes the dynamic at work when payments to hospitals are tied to diagnosis-related groupings (DRGs), a classification or coding system introduced in an effort to control Medicare costs.

Certain codes paid top dollar, so every effort was made to squeeze patients into the higher paying diagnoses. Cardiac catheterization, bypass surgery, and angioplasty paid particularly well, and the number of hospitals performing these procedures increased dramatically. However, since trauma care paid poorly and many trauma patients were uninsured, the number of trauma centers in the country decreased sharply.[35]

Of course the waste produced by this kind of "gaming" activity can also occur in a nonprofit system based on piecework incentives. It happens in Canada to some degree with the fee-for-service system of paying most doctors. In Canadian hospitals, however, public administration has resulted in global budgets that significantly reduce the incentives to emphasize the most complicated and expensive types of care. Under global budgeting, each hospital receives from the province a fixed amount that can then be allocated on the basis of patients' needs rather than on the basis of revenue maximization.

Central to a for-profit system is competition to provide services. Although competition is frequently viewed as a way of increasing efficiency, it too often leads to unnecessary duplication and inefficiency. Competition encourages investment in expensive, sophisticated technologies designed to attract "customers." David Himmelstein and Steffie Woolhandler refer to this as a "medical arms race," resulting in more expensive but not necessarily better care. Reporting on a 1990 study, they show that hospital costs are higher in areas with more competition.[36] As a result, care is not only more costly but also more poorly distributed. Services are concentrated where the returns are highest, among the wealthy and in high-density urban areas. Meanwhile, "those [hospitals] that care for the poor are suffering significant financial losses and closing."[37]

Public administration in Canada, by contrast, makes it possible to provide more equitable distribution while reducing unnecessary duplication.

For example, after adjustment for differences in population size, in 1987 there were 3 times as many hospitals with units providing open-heart surgery in California as in Ontario, 5 times as many with magnetic resonance scanners, and 10 times as many with extracorporeal lithotriptors. One consequence is a much fuller use of capacity in Canada.[38]

Public administration allows for a more rational, holistic assessment of technological requirements, based on evidence about patient needs rather than on marketing considerations.

This leads to yet another reason why costs are higher in for-profit systems. Competition means marketing and marketing means costs. In Canada, the marketing costs in the drug industry are quite striking. This industry spends about $1 billion a year on various forms of product promotion, far outstripping the $89 million it spends on basic research.[39] Much of this promotional activity is aimed directly at patients, who are encouraged to contact their physician about the prescription drug being promoted.[40] Such advertising is a contributing factor in the overutilization and inappropriate use of drugs, thus increasing health care costs.[41] Advertising is limited primarily to the drug industry and to the private supplementary health insurance industry in Canada, because there is little reason for either doctors or hospitals to compete on the open market. As a result, less of the Canadian health dollar is spent on the promotion of particular services.

The drug industry provides a final example of the ways in which for-profit health care can raise costs. It spends large sums not only on sales promotion but also on lobbying governments to secure special treatment and protection. These costs too are passed on to the health care system, in the form of higher drug prices, and to the general public, in the form of tax deductions for lobbying expenses. The lobbying outlays and the tax revenue forgone are much higher in the United States in part because of the presence of many more areas of for-profit activity.[42]

Public Administration, Planning, and Personal Choices

Public administration allows for rational, system-wide planning, individual choice and the exercise of democratic influence in ways that a multi-payer, privately administered system cannot. With a publicly administered yet decentralized system, services can be designed and distributed in ways that combine access with efficiency. And with publicly administered services, individuals and groups can have a vital influence on how health care is delivered, even if sometimes they have to wait until the next election.

Take the case of open-heart surgery, for example. David Naylor, a medical doctor and Rhodes Scholar with a doctoral degree from Oxford in administrative sciences who now directs Ontario's Institute for Clinical Evaluative Sciences, has conducted research on queues for heart surgery in Ontario.[43] Before the case study began, the public plan had used its financial clout to organize the delivery of adult cardiovascular surgery on a regional basis. But in 1989 a Toronto cardiovascular surgeon went to the media with the claim that deaths had occurred on his personal waiting list as a consequence of steadily lengthening queues. The resulting publicity and public pressure prompted the provincial government to appoint a group of providers to develop better mechanisms for ensuring appropriate and timely care.

According to Naylor, the increase in waiting times was real. It was not, however, caused primarily by either cutbacks in funding or a growth in heart disease. Indeed, the incidence of coronary artery disease seemed to be falling. The greater part of the explanation for the growth in waiting lists could be found in two developments. First, physicians were becoming more aggressive about ordering tests, which in turn revealed problems. Second, they were becoming more experienced in conducting the surgery, making it a safer, more effective and thus more attractive technique. This was particularly the case for elderly and high-risk patients, who spent more time in hospital recovery units and thus reduced access for others. In other words, the main cause of the growing waiting lists was to be found in the fact that more and different patients were being recommended for the surgery, rather than reduced resources being devoted to it. The lengthening queues were an indication of the system's success, not of its failure.

The government-launched special investigation into cardiac surgery discovered considerable variation in waiting times and in queuing practices. In response, spot funding was allocated to deal with the bottlenecks and the discrepancies. Nurses were hired and designated to handle the waiting lists in a more organized fashion. Surgeons revised their procedures on the basis of the recommendations arising from the investigation. The result? There was a "dramatic impact" in the length of the queues, which fell by over 40 percent in a year. "Average waiting times were also down dramatically, with elective patients waiting only a few weeks in the hands of most surgeons."[44]

The central lesson from this example is clear. Public administration allowed a prompt response to public pressure that increased individual access to care. And because this access was provided by means of universal public insurance, it was possible to increase it without rationing it on the basis of ability to pay. As Naylor argues,

[q]ueue-based allocation of services, particularly if it is predicated on explicit and objective criteria with selective delay, is potentially superior to price-based rationing, because the latter will almost inevitably lead to implicit and arbitrary denial.[45]

Although a universal and publicly administered plan means that individuals have little or no choice about participating in it or about paying for it through their taxes, this does not mean they have no choices to make. Except in the most isolated areas, individuals can choose which doctors and which hospitals to use, and they can do much more. As the case of cardiovascular surgery in Ontario illustrates, they can influence the overall structure of health care services. They can become active on public bodies such as the boards and committees of public hospitals or of health advocacy groups. And of course they can vote. Because the system is public, it tends to be responsive to strong public pressure.

The choices for individuals are not necessarily greater in a multi-payer system made up of private insurance companies and health care providers. With private insurance plans, often the only choice is to sign up with another plan, and even this choice is often made by the employer, not by the individual. A 1996 survey of more than 1,000 large firms in the United States found that 47 percent "offered only one health plan in 1996, a rise from 41 percent in 1995."[46] Although public administration may not always be easy to influence, individuals and groups are more likely to have an impact on it than they are on the giant, multinational corporations that increasingly dominate the private health care system.

Conclusion

Public administration in health care does not mean endless regulations, limitations, and bureaucracy. Nor does it significantly reduce choices, compared to the private health insurance alternatives. What the evidence shows is that public administration reduces costs and allows for the delivery of quality health care in accessible fashion based on health needs.

7

A Perfect System?

Is Canada's single-payer health care system perfect? Of course not. But it has been improved in a variety of ways since its inception, and the fact that it is paid for by public insurance makes it more sensitive to public opinion than are systems based on the profit motive. Problems remain, but they are not those commonly cited by media and other critics of public health insurance. It is to the problems, imagined and real, of Canadian medicare that we now turn.

What the Problems Are Not

I. Finances

Comparisons of public spending in Canada and other industrialized countries show two things. The Canadian level of public expenditure is in line with levels elsewhere, and it is very much under control. These conclusions hold, however public spending is measured.

Critics have argued that the Canadian public system spends both too much and too little on health care. At the height of the debt and deficit hysteria that swept through Canada, all social programs came under attack. These programs, including health care, were blamed for causing the debt through profligate overspending.

The charge did not stand up to careful scrutiny, however. In an

Table 7.1
PUBLIC SPENDING ON HEALTH CARE
SELECTED INDUSTRIALIZED COUNTRIES

Country	Percentage of GDP 1995	Percentage of all public spending, 1994*
Germany	8.2	18.4
France	7.7	13.6
Switzerland	7.1	18.6
Belgium	7.0	12.6
Canada	6.9	14.5
Iceland	6.9	17.7
Netherlands	6.8	12.2
United States	6.6	16.4

*The figure for Iceland's percentage of all public spending refers to 1995; for the United States it refers to 1993.

Source: Organisation for Economic Co-operation and Development, "OECD Health Data 97." http"//www.oecd.org/statlist.htm (updated July 8, 1997), Health I Table.

analysis published by Statistics Canada's leading economic journal, two highly respected economists demonstrated that the growth in spending on all social programs, indeed on all programs, accounted for virtually none of the federal debt accumulated by the late 1980s. Rather, the debt was primarily attributable to a combination of reductions in corporate taxes and increases in real interest rates, or to the cost to the government (and others) of borrowing money.[1] Spending on social programs in general, and on health care in particular, is not the problem.

Some U.S. critics of the Canadian health care system have claimed that it is too expensive in light of the heavy tax burden it creates. Like health care spending, however, the level of taxes in Canada is about average in comparison with the levels in other industrialized countries. Both Canadian payroll taxes and fringe benefit costs are among the lowest, in large measure because of Canada's public, universal and quite comprehensive health care system. Moreover, as the *World Competitiveness Report 1991* pointed out, publicly funded health care was a major factor placing Canada as high as fifth in its world competitiveness rankings.[2]

At the same time, some critics on both sides of the border have argued that on certain items Canada spends too little to provide adequate care. There is, however, little evidence that spending more would result in better or more accessible care. When public and private spending are combined, Canada spends much less on health care than the United States. Yet for less money, Canada provides more hospital beds relative to population and the average lengths of stay in its hospitals are longer. The United States does have slightly more doctors, and many more of its doctors are specialists, but there is research to indicate that this represents excess capacity more than it represents what is needed for quality care.[3] In the midst of American plenty, moreover, there remain considerable shortages because the private system in the United States has greater difficulty distributing care equitably and efficiently. A 1996 study found that "problems in getting needed medical care affect about 17 million uninsured adults and 17 million insured adults in America."[4] This happens to very few Canadians.

There is no way to determine scientifically the appropriate amount to spend on health care. The allocation of society's resources is as much a matter of values as it is of evidence. For their part, Canadians have made it abundantly clear that they want to continue to devote a significant proportion of their tax dollars to health care. Canadians do not feel that they spend too much on their medicare system. Nor do they feel that they receive inadequate returns on their investment.

II. Waiting Lists

The rich cannot buy their way to the front of the line in the Canadian health care system. A few of them, and some U.S. critics, have as a result taken to complaining about the delays experienced before certain procedures are carried out. There are several aspects of the waiting list issue that merit consideration.

First, every society is almost certain to impose at least some waiting time for some health care procedures on at least some of its members. Every country in the world, including both Canada and the United States, does so now and always has. To do otherwise would be possible, after enough providers were trained and facilities built, but it would be done at the cost of other priorities, including those that affect the social determinants of health. Just as one would not build the capacity of a mass transit system so that everyone has a comfortable seat during rush hour, so too with health care. The issue is not whether there should be rationing and waiting, but the principles that should govern the rationing and waiting.

Second, it should be made crystal clear that Canadians rarely wait for care that is required immediately. And, given that there are no financial costs to the individual at the point of receiving care, there is little incentive for patients to wait until their problems are severe. Most of the reports on waiting times that circulate widely refer to elective surgery, not to care that is required immediately.

Third, it should be remembered that Canadians have become so accustomed to readily accessible care that is portable throughout the country and that comes without cost to the individual that any waiting is considered intolerable. Surveys suggesting that waiting times have increased may thus leave a misleading impression. They may refer to increases in waiting times from a very low base, rather than the actual time people have to wait.

Fourth, we have scant comparative data in Canada, or in other countries, that would provide a solid basis for assessing the actual amounts of time people wait for care, or the consequences of their waits. How long, for example, do the "working poor" in the United States wait for diabetes diagnosis or for cataract surgery? In Canada, does waiting for elective surgery have long-term negative consequences? What are the consequences of waiting for different kinds of elective surgery? No discussion of waiting times can be adequate without such information.

Finally, and perhaps most importantly, the example of cardiac surgery in Ontario demonstrates that public systems are in a position to address waiting list problems when they are revealed. As the National Forum on Health explains,

Experience . . . suggests that public health care can reduce waiting lists without increasing spending. The key is to ensure that waiting lists are structured and prioritized, and that incentives are in place to ensure that patients are served before their risk, or their degree of suffering, becomes unacceptably high. The solution is management, monitoring, and evaluation—not a bewildering array of public and private alternatives.[5]

III. Bureaucracy and Privacy

The beauty of the Canadian system lies in its simplicity. First, there were two short pieces of legislation, one on hospital insurance and then another on physician insurance. In 1984, these were consolidated and expanded into the Canada Health Act, another short and simple piece of legislation. Basically, the Canada Health Act lays down the five principles for the federal contribution to the funding of provincial health care programs. It therefore allows for diversity among and within provinces without creating enormous amounts of surveillance work. Health services have remained largely the way they were before medicare, except that now the bills are sent to a single payer in each province.

The consequence is less bureaucracy for both providers and patients. Because everyone belongs to the system, there is no need for fat files on each individual. Because the bills are paid from one source with little hassle, there is no need for detailed accounts of the supplies and services used by individuals, no need to hire collection agencies, and few resources spent on court battles over liability.

When Tommy Douglas first proposed to introduce public insurance coverage for doctors' services, one of the specters raised by his political opponents was that the confidentiality of individual health records would be lost. Public insurance was equated with government snooping into everyone's health file.

Ironically, however, personal health records and other personal records are much more likely to be invaded by private insurance companies competing to avoid high risks than by the public insurance agency. With everyone enrolled in a universal public scheme, there is no need to check individual medical histories or any other personal information to decide on program eligibility. And with everyone enrolled, there is also no reason to check on credit ratings, or on employment histories and status. Neither patients nor providers need to gain prior approval before undergoing tests or treatments, thus further reducing the situations in which outsiders demand personal health information. With hospitals operating under global budgets within a universal scheme, there is no need for financial administrators inside or outside the hospital to examine individual patient files.

All this contrasts sharply with private health insurance schemes. Private insurers have a financial incentive not only to enroll the best risks but also to specify as precisely as possible the services to be covered. A family history of cancer, a gay lifestyle, a clearly dangerous job or high job turnover could all mean a person is a risk. To make their enrollment and coverage decisions, private insurers need access to detailed personal medical, financial, and employment histories; to test results; and to physician and hospital practice patterns. Not incidently, they also need detailed reports on what individual physicians do, so their risk of incurring costs can be assessed. These requirements mean more bureaucracy and less privacy.

Drug prescription records may appear to provide an exception to the general rule thats a public system protects privacy better. In Ontario, for example, the government has funded the establishment of a computer network that allows pharmacists to coordinate personal records on the filling of drug prescriptions. This integrated computer system enables pharmacists to watch out for drugs that may interact in harmful ways and for drugs that may be over-prescribed. The system could also enable the public insurance agency to monitor the prescribing patterns of individual doctors and the prescription drugs purchased by individual patients. It has been set up, however, on a voluntary basis, and the government and its public health insurance agency have no privileged access to individual prescription drug records.

What a public system does allow for is more information on, and more choice about, who has access to information on individual health files and on provider patterns. Again to use the example of Ontario, patient rights advocates have successfully pressed for legislation that severely restricts access to personal information on the diagnosis and treatment of mental illness. Not even parents and other relatives responsible for providing care, let alone insurance companies and governments, have access to the files without the permission of the adult patient.

IV. Choices and Abuses

Unlike the United States, which funds individuals who meet predetermined criteria, Canada has decided to fund services for everyone through a public system. As a result, Canadians have many more health care choices than do Americans. They are not prevented by predetermined criteria from qualifying for care. Individual Canadian patients and family physicians choose without outside interference who will be seen how often and by whom. On referral from a family physician, Canadian patients can go to any specialist or hospital, as frequently as medically appropriate and for as long as medically necessary.

Doctors too enjoy a wide range of choices, and freedom from supervision. There is little restriction on where they locate. In fact, a recent court decision in British Columbia struck down a provision in the fee schedule that penalized new entrants to medicine if they chose to set up their practices in heavily served urban areas. In this instance, the problem appears to be too much individual choice in the public system, not too little.[6] Physicians are guaranteed that their fees will be paid at the negotiated rate, and only very seldom are their activities scrutinized. Usually the monitoring of physicians' fees simply takes the form of letters sent to a random sample of patients inquiring whether they visited a specific physician on a specific date. The fee-for-service system under which nine out of ten Canadian doctors are paid allows them considerable choice about their hours of work and, ultimately, about how much income they will receive.

Like doctors, nurses and most other care providers in the public system must meet the health profession's standards of their province in order to practice in it. Most of the many female care providers are unionized, improving their choices in terms of pay, benefits, and working conditions.[7] The stability of a publicly financed system has been an important factor in this high rate of unionization.

The other side of choice is abuse. Within Canada, the claim is at times made that patients overuse their system, abusing their right to free choice and "free" care. This complaint is frequently combined with a call for user fees. The argument is advanced that such fees would simultaneously make people appreciate the benefits of the system more and make them be more careful about using it, thus ensuring more appropriate utilization.

There is very little evidence, however, of widespread abuse of access to care by Canadians. Nor is there evidence that user fees would prevent any of the abuse that does exist. One difficulty with attempting to collect such evidence concerns the definition of abuse. Those who use the system are unlikely to think that they are abusing it. Ask any patient waiting in a hospital emergency room, painfully or anxiously, whether *others* are there for frivolous reasons. Many will say that others do not look like they need immediate care. But they will be firmly convinced that their own visit is urgent and justified.

Furthermore, much of what might be defined as inappropriate use of the system would be so defined *after* diagnosis. Hindsight has 20/20 vision, as the saying goes. A mother may rush her screaming child to emergency only to discover that the problem is an earache that could have been dealt with by the family physician during regular office hours. But the earache could also have been an indication of a much more serious condition, and urgent care was sought precisely to find this out. When abuse is defined as use that is not medically necessary, the research that does exist has found very little abuse by patients.[8]

As a team of Canadian researchers has concluded from a thorough analysis of the uses of user fees,

it is difficult to see how *patient*-initiated abuse *could* make up a large share of overall health care use and costs, because patients have little control over most of the decisions about the use of care. Call-back visits, referrals, hospital admissions and prescriptions, for example, all depend on the judgment and approval of a physician. No doubt there are some patients who "demand" a hospital procedure or a prescription, but the picture of patients eagerly requesting surgery or wanting to take medication just because the services are "free" makes even advocates of user charges laugh.[9]

At the same time, there is some evidence that the public insurance system encourages appropriate use in Canada. A study by Kevin Gorey published in a 1997 issue of the *American Journal of Public Health* found that "compared to their Detroit counterparts, poor women in Toronto have a survival rate for breast cancer that is 30 percent higher, for ovarian cancer that is 38 percent higher and for cervical cancer that is 48 percent higher." Moreover, "Toronto women have survival rates more than 50 percent above that of women in Detroit's poorest districts for lung, stomach and pancreatic cancer." Even after accounting for race and for the standards for measuring poverty, the differences remain.[10] The research suggests that Canadian medicare, with no user charges at the point of service, encourages appropriate and timely use, while user charges and other provisions that limit choice make the U.S. health care system less effective.

V. Quality, Technology, Research, and Innovation

Although it must be conceded that the Canadian system is more equitable than the U.S. alternative, it is on occasion argued that the quality of care is inferior in Canada, especially when it comes to advances related to research and technology. As we have seen, measuring quality is no simple task, and neither country is very good at it. Too much of the research on both sides of the border focuses on costs, measuring quality in terms of dollars spent and efficiency in terms of dollars saved. On both sides of the border, we know much more about expenditures per person than we do about whether these expenditures are worthwhile in terms of health outcomes.

As a result, researchers in both Canada and the United States have turned increasingly to the development of new and better ways to assess the quality of the care that is delivered. Especially for a country with a small population, Canada has a significant number of research organizations devoted to the assessment of quality in the delivery of health services. There are, for example, major centers at several universities in the provinces of British Columbia, Ontario, and Quebec that bring together multidisciplinary teams to examine health policy issues. The province of Manitoba has a Centre for Health Policy and Evaluation that maintains a database for hospital discharge information, enabling it to assess both the accessibility and the quality of care. Ontario's Institute for Clinical Evaluative Sciences (ICES) regularly produces a practice atlas that documents variations in practice patterns across the province, in an effort to prompt medical and other practitioners to evaluate whether they are following the most appropriate procedures. The Saskatchewan Health Services Utilization Review Commission (HSURC) has conducted and publicized a wide range of studies to help providers decide on the best approaches to care.

These and similar research organizations receive the bulk of their funding from the public purse. There are also national and provincial granting councils that provide financial support to individual researchers and teams of researchers based in hospitals and universities in every part of the country.[11] Lesser amounts come from a variety of charitable foundations. Partly as a result of this tax-supported investment in research, Canadians proportionately publish virtually as many articles in medical journals as do their U.S. counterparts.[12]

All this research activity leads to a number of conclusions. First, Canada devotes considerable time and resources to health-related research, and this research is frequently the basis for innovations in practice. Second, none of the research on quality reveals the existence of significant differences in the quality of health care in Canada and the United States. Although there is relatively more technology in the U.S., there is little evidence to show that all this technology is necessary or related to better quality care. There is, however, evidence that Canada distributes its technology more appropriately and equitably. Third, although neither country has developed very rigorous ways of measuring quality, the establishment of well-funded research centers in Canada with mandates to focus on evaluation and utilization concerns may bode well for the future.[13] The existence of a publicly administered health care system in Canada enhances the likelihood that research conducted there and abroad will be translated into improved care.

133

What the Problems Are

I. Drugs

Canada does have a problem with drugs. Per capita spending on drugs increased by over 100 percent in real terms between 1975 and 1996, rising to $C 362 for every man, woman and child. Drugs now account for over 14 percent of all health care expenditures, virtually the same amount as that spent on physicians and second only to hospitals in terms of expenditure share.[14]

There are three major reasons for this dramatic increase in the amount spent on drugs. First, only three provinces have universal drug plans, and only British Columbia uses a reference-based pricing scheme to help control costs. In its first ten months of operation, British Columbia saved an estimated $21 million by generally paying for only the lowest cost drug in each of three designated "therapeutic categories."[15] In consultation with physicians and pharmacists, the province is working to introduce more therapeutic categories to the scheme, but other provinces have not to date introduced similar approaches. Those provinces without universal plans have multi-payer systems that are comparable to those prevailing in the United States. With such systems, not only are many individuals left out, especially among the "working poor," but it is very difficult for any particular plan to control costs. At the same time, each of them faces unnecessarily high administrative costs.

Second, the Canadian government has in recent years provided special status to the brand-name pharmaceutical firms, protecting them from competition. In the early years of medicare, the government had taken steps to control drug costs through a "compulsory licensing" policy. Compulsory licensing allowed the importing, manufacture, sale, and use of generic copies of the brand-name drugs before their patents expired. In return for receiving licenses from the Commissioner of Patents, the generic drug companies paid royalties to the patent holders. According to a 1985 report, this policy encouraged competition and lowered prices, while still providing healthy profits to the brand-name companies holding the patents.[16]

134

The end of compulsory licensing began in 1987 with an amendment to the Patent Act forbidding generic copies for ten years after the brand-name drug came onto the market. This was followed in 1993 by the Patent Act Amendment Act, commonly referred to as Bill C-91. By extending the protection against generic copies for at least twenty years, Bill C-91 effectively ended compulsory licensing. Reporting on its extensive discussion group sessions, the National Forum on Health concluded that the Canadian public recognize that the intended effect of Bill-C91, "as with any patent legislation, is to limit competition and raise prices, and industry profits." The Forum also found that Canadians were quite skeptical about the promised benefits from this monopoly, benefits such as new and better drugs that would improve health outcomes and reduce the cost of care in the long run.[17]

This leads to the third reason for spiraling drug costs—the increasing reliance on drug therapy, especially expensive drug therapy. Some of the new drugs have made it possible for patients to leave the hospital earlier or to avoid admission altogether. Others have prolonged life and relieved pain. There is, however, considerable evidence that many of the new drugs are neither necessary nor necessarily expensive. Drugs are all too frequently over-used or inappropriately used.[18] And with more money spent by the drug companies on promotion than on research and more on dividends than on production, prices do not reflect what it costs to develop, manufacture and distribute the drugs we now have or will have.

It is primarily for these reasons in 1996 that the National Forum on Health recommended in its final report that Canada "move toward integration of prescription drugs as a fully funded component of publicly funded health care."[19] In the National Forum's view, this universal drug scheme should be supplemented by a comprehensive, publicly run drug information system. It also strongly opposed the direct marketing of prescription drugs to consumers. Although it recognized that the patent legislation could limit the impact of these and other efforts at cost control, it nonetheless settled for recommending only that Bill C-91 be amended to require that drug companies provide additional funding for health research, broadly defined. The Forum did recognize that research funded by drug companies does not always represent the most objective scientific research or the best public interest. It was therefore also recommended that these research funds be administered by the national research granting agencies at full arm's length from the drug industry and following a normal peer-reviewed process. As this set of recommendations demonstrates, there is room in the Canadian system for improvement, and room for public discussion on how to achieve it.

II. Fee-for-Service Payments

The fee-for-service system by which most Canadian doctors are paid creates a second problem area. Payment on this piecework basis, especially when some of the pieces are rewarded much more handsomely than others, contains a built-in incentive to provide more, and more expensive, treatment. This not only inflates the amounts spent on doctors. It also translates into higher overall costs because it is the doctors who control entry to hospitals and to a wide range of other services. Equally important, some of these services may be unnecessary or even dangerous. A much higher proportion of Canadian doctors are paid on a fee-for-service basis than is the case in the United States and this greater reliance on fee for service may translate into excess costs and too much care.[20]

Experience with doctors employed by clinics in the provinces of Saskatchewan and Ontario has demonstrated that these salaried doctors order fewer, and less complicated, treatments overall. They also spend more time with each patient, especially on issues related to health promotion.[21] In spite of this evidence, Canada has taken only a few tentative steps towards increasing the number of salaried doctors. Although many of their members, especially in emergency room work, family practices, and academic settings, would prefer to be salaried, organized medicine remains strongly opposed.

One approach gaining currency in Canada is the idea of paying doctors, and in particular family physicians grouped into primary care organizations, on a capitation basis. Rather than being paid a set fee per service, they would be paid a set fee per patient, and would be responsible for ensuring that their patients received all necessary care, except perhaps for the most elaborate hospital services. Patients would be required to sign up, or "roster," with a particular doctor or group of doctors who would then provide all primary care and control entry to the entire range of health services. This payment method is modeled on practices found in many U.S. health maintenance organizations, where it has been introduced primarily as a cost-cutting strategy.[22]

Capitation could easily undermine most or all of the principles of the Canada Health Act, however. Experience with capitation in the United States shows that this payment method may save some money but, especially in for-profit settings, it often does so at the expense of all that Canadians value in their health care system.

Portability could be severely restricted if patients were limited to the doctor or doctors with whom they were rostered. Comprehensiveness could be impeded by the single entry point, if the gatekeepers get to earn more by referring their patients for fewer services. While fee-for-service contains the "perverse incentive" of promoting over-utilization, capitation contains the opposite perverse incentive, promoting under-utilization. This could in turn further reduce accessibility, another of medicare's five principles. And, if primary care organizations were allowed or required to establish their own recruitment and enrollment procedures, accessibility could also be threatened by "cherry picking" or "skimming" strategies, as organizations competed to attract the healthiest members, to whom they could then offer the best services at the lowest cost. A few persons with HIV/AIDS could absorb the entire budget of a small organization funded through capitation. In the United States, patients with poor medical histories or poor genes can find it difficult to enroll in for-profit schemes. In the process, universality could be undermined, as particularly vulnerable groups such as the homeless and the illiterate fail to get signed up with a primary care practice. And in the end, care might be more expensive as it is in the United States.

All Canadians are already signed up with one of the provincial plans. If everyone had to sign up with a primary care organization which received its revenue from capitation, the administrative costs to medicare would soar. The Saskatchewan and Ontario clinics, and the Quebec social service centers (CLSCs), with their global budgets and

137

salaried staff, including doctors, provide far better models for payment, models that support and strengthen the principles of the Canada Health Act.

III. Privatization

Like other countries around the world, Canada has become increasingly concerned about the levels of health expenditure and increasingly interested in reforms that promise to deliver more effective, efficient care.[23] And, like many other countries, Canada has turned to the private, for-profit sector for models to emulate. This is especially the case with practices developed in the United States.

The reliance on private-sector practices is based on two assumptions, or what might better be termed articles of faith, given that there is scant evidence to back them up. One of these assumptions is that, because they have to operate in competitive markets where consumer choice prevails, private-sector firms are necessarily more efficient and effective than public-sector organizations. The second, related assumption is that health care can be readily transformed into a free, competitive market like the rest.[24] It follows from these assumptions that private-sector practices will necessarily work in health care. Both of these assumptions can be challenged, and challenged on the basis of experience in the United States.

The stage for privatization was set in Canada by a growing concern among politicians and in the business community over the public debt, and a growing fear in the population that the public debt would mean that their health care system would disappear unless reforms were instituted. The increasingly explicit faith shown by public policy makers in private-sector methods,[25] combined with significant pressure from firms seeking to profit from Canadian health care, have led to more and more privatization in the system. This privatization has taken a number of forms.

One form can be found particularly within the hospital sector. Here administrations faced with constantly shrinking budgets have looked to private-sector management practices as a way to reduce costs. Total Quality Management (TQM), or some variant of this approach, has become increasingly popular. It has been embraced by both the National Forum on Health and the agency that accredits Canadian hospitals. Philip Hassen, the former chief executive officer of a major Ontario teaching hospital, went so far in his enthusiasm to assert that this model, developed in the Japanese and then U.S. auto industries, is even more applicable to health care. He holds this view "because total quality management, like health care, claims to be based on concepts of service, commitment and continuous quality improvement, as well as teamwork in everything."[26]

Teamwork is intimately related to multi-skilling and this practice in particular has been attractive to hospital administrators. It also provides a very clear example of what is problematic in using car-manufacturing strategies for care delivery. Multi-skilling, in its best form, means a team works together to get a project done. It also means that one worker can be substituted for another when a member is absent for some reason, and that all employees can take up any task on demand, in an effort to avoid wasted time. This may work in a factory, where job components have been broken down into easily learned parts. In a hospital, however, much of the work involves highly skilled providers with specialized knowledge whose jobs require both a grasp of complex interactions and an appreciation of whole people. Yet some hospitals have been following private-sector strategies in substituting less skilled providers for more skilled ones on these teams. As is the case in the United States, some Canadian nurses are seeing their jobs subdivided and handed over to workers with minimal training. The consequences of asking a housekeeper to sterilize equipment in the operating room may not be immediately obvious, but a more careful consideration will make it clear that it can be very problematic to have untrained people in such a critical environment where every action counts.[27]

Central to these private-sector management strategies is management control through measurement. What counts is what can be counted. "If you can't measure it, you can't manage it" is a truism in new management theory, one that is favorably cited in a recent report to the Canadian Deputy Ministers of Health.[28] More and more hospitals are buying technology developed in the United States to measure work, processes, and outcomes. While some measurement is obviously useful, many of the significant aspects of care cannot be easily counted or measured. Take the case of changing a bed. The length of time it will take in a hospital will vary considerably with the particular equipment involved in the patient's care, with the patient's capacity, with the number and skills of the team members providing the care, and with the patient's need for comfort and support. Emotional support in particular is difficult to measure, but so too is the entire bed-making process. This is particularly the case if the goal is to provide care and not just to change sheets.

These measures are often used to develop formulas for the time required for care. Here, too, Canadian hospitals have looked to U.S. models in shortening patient stays and switching to day surgery for a growing number of operations. Again, these strategies may have some uses, but they too often lead to one formula for the infinite variety of people requiring care. Childbirth provides just one example. In the United States, legislation has been introduced in several states to allow women giving birth to stay longer than the twenty-four hours allowed by many managed care plans, if more time is necessary. The legislation was required precisely because when formulas are universally applied, some patients do not have their needs for care met and some patients are put at risk.

In addition to adopting private-sector management practices, hospitals have also been contracting out more of their services to for-profit concerns. This form of privatization not only assumes that the private sector can naturally provide cheaper and more effective care, but also that certain aspects of service delivery can be readily separated out from care delivery. Services contracted out more frequently are then often referred to as "hotel services," another practice adopted from the United States.

Yet those who drafted the Canadian legislation setting up hospital insurance included food, cleaning, and other services as part of the package. Their inclusion of these as elements of care is very much in keeping with the current research in health, which demonstrates that nutrition, sanitation, and properly maintained facilities are central to health. Indeed, they are even more important to those who are ill and therefore particularly vulnerable. Contracting out these services as "hotel services" implies that no special skills are required to support the sick at the same time as it denies the role these services play in health. Preliminary research in Canada suggests moreover that contracted out services are neither cheaper nor as safe as those provided by hospital employees.

When hospitals move to day surgery, outpatient services, and shorter patient stays, they are privatizing care in another way. Patients, and the cost of their care, are largely shifted to the private household. The Canadian health care system takes up some of the responsibility for this care through home care services.[29] But as the women in particular who were surveyed for the National Forum on Health made clear, most of the work is left to women at home, which means that more of the costs are shifted to the household. The Forum's response was to recommend further data collection to determine the degree to which care has been off-loaded to women working without pay at home.[30]

Yet many Canadians indicated to the National Forum that much more is required to ensure that the five principles are upheld as care delivery is restructured. For one thing, drugs and other supplies that are provided without charge in the hospital often need to be provided to the patient in the home through private means. There is growing pressure across the country to provide more, and more comprehensive, services that recognize the extent to which care has been moved into the home.

The National Forum heard from a large number of women that home care meant that they were being "conscripted" into care work. And many were conscientious objectors to this new form of conscription. In response, the Forum recommended the further extension of public insurance to cover more home care needs. But more home care may simply mean that women have a few more hours free from conscripted service. Without adequate alternatives in a variety of institutional settings, and without the assurance that care will be provided by people with the required skills, more publicly funded home care will not be enough to keep women, and those they care for, healthy.

With a new commitment to small government has come further cutbacks in health spending at all levels. The cuts are justified as necessary because of the debt as well as desirable because they will make health care more effective. The benefits have so far failed to appear, however, and most Canadians see instead a reduction in services and a threat to their beloved health care system. That these strategies taken from the for-profit sector have not helped individuals is evident in the significant growth in private health spending in recent years. Private spending, which was stabilized at about a quarter of all Canadian health expenditures until 1992, accounted for 30 percent of all spending in 1996.[31] The fact that private spending rises as public-sector spending falls suggests that many of these services were necessary, and that privatization strategies are more likely to mean that the individual pays rather than that the costs of care are reduced.

These changes were not made necessary by overspending on health or by grossly inefficient services. And certainly the American mainly private system has not fared better in terms of either cost or efficiency. Reform strategies in the United States are receiving even less favor. Indeed, a 1997 poll classifying industries according to how good a job they were doing, found "health insurance companies and managed-care companies were ranked second and third from the bottom (just above the tobacco industry)."[32] It is therefore difficult to see why it should provide a model for reform. A 1985 study by the federal government's Health and Welfare Canada concluded that "the often asserted benefits of privatization were largely absent, or were unknown and possibly suspect."[33] Yet as individual costs rise and services are reduced with funding cutbacks and private-sector practices, there is increasing demand from some groups for more private, for-profit care. While this may not have been the conscious objective of the cutbacks, it certainly has been the effect.

What is a major problem for the Canadian system then is not bureaucracy, rising costs, waiting lists, or poor quality care. If anything, these problems are arising as a consequence of strategies for reform, of a move to a more private, multi-payer approach to health care.

Conclusion

The Canadian health care system provides universal, accessible portable, comprehensive care at reasonable cost through a public insurance system. This system separates purchasers and providers, with the public insurance scheme paying for services provided by others. This provincially administered system allows flexibility as well as choices for patients and providers. At the same time it permits planning to avoid unnecessary duplication and limitation on access.

The Canadian system is neither free of flaws nor fixed in time. It is evolving in response to new developments in health care research and to new political pressures. The popular support for it nevertheless remains wide and deep. It enjoys more support from its citizens than can be claimed by the health care systems in other countries. For Canada, and for Canadians, medicare works.

Notes

CHAPTER 1. A CANADIAN LOVE AFFAIR

1. These results come from a 1993 Gallup poll cited in Nicole Nolan, "Bitter Medicine," *In These Times* (Jan. 20, 1997), p. 16.

2. National Forum on Health, "Values Working Group Synthesis Report," *Canada Health Action: Building on the Legacy,* Vol. II, *Synthesis Reports and Issues Papers* (Ottawa: Minister of Public Works and Government Services, 1997), p. 5.

3. National Forum on Health, "Values Working Group," p. 11.

4. Frank Graves, "Canadian Health Care—What Are the Facts? An Overview of Public Opinion in Canada," in *Access to Quality Health Care for All Canadians* (Ottawa: Canadian Medical Association, 1996), pp. 18–19.

5. In *Maclean's* (Dec. 2, 1996), pp. 50–51.

6. *UC Berkeley Wellness Newsletter* (May 1997).

7. Quoted in Malcolm G. Taylor, *Health Insurance and Canadian Public Policy: The Seven Decisions That Created the Canadian Health Insurance System and Their Consequences,* 2nd ed. (Kingston and Montreal: McGill-Queen's University Press, 1989), p. 433.

8. To borrow the titles from two books on Canadian approaches to the organization of social services: C. David Naylor, *Private Practices, Public Payment: Canadian Medicine and the Politics of Health Insurance 1911–1966* (Kingston: McGill–Queen's University Press, 1986); Josephine Rekart, *Public Funds, Private Provision* (Vancouver: University of British Columbia Press, 1994).

9. Robert Evans, "Health Care Reform: 'The Issue From Hell'," *Policy Options* (July–Aug. 1993), p. 37 (emphasis in original).

10. David U. Himmelstein and Steffie Woolhandler, *The National Health Program Book* (Monroe, ME: Common Courage Press, 1994), p. 40.

11. Robert J. Blendon and Humphrey Taylor, "Views on Health Care: Public Opinion in Three Nations," *Health Affairs* 8:1 (spring 1989), p. 152, where it is reported that 61 percent of Americans "would prefer the Canadian system of national health insurance" to the system they have now.

CHAPTER 2. HOW CANADIANS GOT UNIVERSAL COVERAGE

1. Doris Shackleton, *Tommy Douglas* (Toronto: McClelland and Stewart, 1975), p. 17.

2. See Malcolm G. Taylor, *Health Insurance and Canadian Public Policy,* 2nd ed. (Kingston and Montreal: McGill–Queen's University Press, 1987); G. Harvey Agnew, *Canadian Hospitals 1920 to 1970: A Dramatic Half Century* (Toronto: University of Toronto Press, 1974); and Paul Starr, "Transformations in Defeat: The Changing Objectives of National Health Insurance, 1915–1980," *American Journal of Public Health* 72 (1982), pp. 78–88.

3. See Helen Heeney and Susan Charters, *Life Before Medicare: Canadian Experiences* (Toronto: The Stories Project, 1995).

4. Taylor, *Health Insurance,* p. 2.

5. Quoted in Taylor, *Health Insurance,* p. 80.

6. See Taylor, *Health Insurance,* p. 104. This discussion of Saskatchewan relies heavily on Taylor's account.

7. Taylor, *Health Insurance,* p. 111.

8. Taylor, *Health Insurance,* p. 113.

9. See Taylor, *Health Insurance,* p. 114.

10. Quoted in Taylor, *Health Insurance,* p. 223.

11. At 36.2 percent, the largest five-year increase in patient days in public general and allied special hospitals occurred between 1950 and 1955. During the 1955–60 period, when public hospital insurance was introduced, the increase in patient days fell to 22.5 percent, and the rate of increase kept falling in subsequent periods. Calculated from F. H. Leacy, ed., *Historical Statistics of Canada,* 2nd ed. (Ottawa: Minister of Supply and Services Canada for Statistics Canada, 1983), Series B 192.

12. Pat Armstrong et al, *Vital Signs: Nursing in Transition* (Toronto: Garamond Press, 1993), p. 38.
13. For excellent coverage of this strike see the documentary film, *Bitter Medicine: Part One, The Birth of Medicare*, (Montreal: National Film Board of Canada, 1983).
14. Taylor, *Health Insurance*, p. 329.
15. This quote is taken from a report on a conference held to bring together the CMA and the organization representing the insurance companies. The report was made by a former executive director of Trans-Canada Medical Services, C. Howard Shillington, in his book *Road To Medicare* (Toronto: Del Graphics, 1972), pp. 140–41.
16. John K. Iglehart, "Physicians and the Growth of Managed Care," *New England Journal of Medicine* 331:17 (Oct. 27, 1994), p. 1167. See also, for example, Marsha R. Gold et al, "A National Survey of the Arrangements Managed-Care Plans Make with Physicians," *New England Journal of Medicine* 333:25 (Dec. 21, 1995); Gordon Schiff, "Why for-profit managed care fails you and your patients," *ACP Observer* (American College of Physicians) 16:10 (Nov. 1996); Lloyd I. Sederer and Steven M. Mirin, "The Impact of Managed Care on Clinical Practice," *Psychiatric Quarterly* 65:3 (fall 1994); or, in a more popular vein, William Sherman, "Health: Mismanaged Care," *Vogue* (Feb. 1996).
17. Cited in Taylor, *Health Insurance*, p. 367.
18. See Stephen J. Kunitz, "Socialism and Social Insurance in the United States and Canada," pp.104–24 in C. David Naylor, ed., *Canadian Health Care and the State* (Kingston and Montreal: McGill–Queen's University Press, 1992), p. 112.
19. World Economic Forum, *World Competitiveness Report 1991* (Lausanne, Switzerland: Institut pour l'étude des methodes de direction de l'entreprise, 1992).
20. David U. Himmelstein and Steffie Woolhandler, *The National Health Program Book* (Monroe, ME: Common Courage Press, 1994), p. 40.
21. Charles Andrews, *Profit Fever: The Drive to Corporatize Health Care and How to Stop It* (Monroe, ME: Common Courage Press, 1995), p. 90, citing Neil Rolde, *Your Money or Your Health* (New York: Paragon House, 1992), p. 7.
22. Monique Bégin, *Medicare: Canada's Right to Health,* David Homel and Lucille Nelson, trans. (Montreal: Optimum Publishing, 1988), p. 27.
23. Philip E. Enterline et al, "Effects of 'Free' Medical Care on Medical Prac-

tice: The Quebec Experience," *New England Journal of Medicine* 288:2 (May 31, 1973).

24. Bernard R. Blishen, *Doctors in Canada: The Changing World of Medical Practice* (Toronto: University of Toronto Press in association with Statistics Canada, 1991), tables 3.7 and 3.11. Includes only active civilian physicians and excludes interns and residents.

25. Bégin, *Medicare*, pp. 9–10.

26. Bégin, *Medicare*, p. 93.

27. Bégin, *Medicare*, p. 126.

28. E. M. Hall, *Canada's National-Provincial Health Program for the 1980s* (Ottawa: Health and Welfare Canada, 1980).

29. Canada Health Act, 1984, c.6. Preamble.

30. Canada Health Act, 1984, c.6.s.3

31. Canada Health Act, 1984, c.6. Preamble.

CHAPTER 3. GETTING ACCESS

1. Cited in Jeanne Kessler, *Bitter Medicine* (New York: Birch Lane Press, 1994), p. 19.

2. Monique Bégin, *Medicare: Canada's Right to Health,* David Homel and Lucille Nelson, trans. (Montreal: Optimum Publishing, 1988), p. 25.

3. According to a recent newspaper article by Anthony DePalma, ("Doctor, What's the Prognosis? A Crisis for Canada," *New York Times,* Dec. 15, 1996), Canadians are being forced to "accept far less than the best" because of long waiting lists, the absence of some sophisticated technologies, and an exodus over the last four years of about 4 percent of the nation's doctors, mostly to the United States. DePalma's sources, however, were primarily doctors in Ontario at a time when their agreement with the provincial government was in dispute, and he did have to acknowledge that Canadians continue to reject proposals to make their system more like that in the United States. His specific criticisms are taken up later in this chapter. Meanwhile, part of the explanation for the overwhelming preference expressed by Canadians for their own system may be found in a report from another U.S. journalist, William C. Symonds ("Whither a Health-Care Solution? Oh, Canada" and "From Canada, A Satisfied Customer Reports" *Business Week,* Mar. 21, 1994). According to Symonds, Canada's single-payer system is "by far the best way to control costs while

preserving the freedom of choice and physician autonomy that made American medicine great." The system's "quality of care is still exceptionally high," he argued.

4. See the Canada Health Act, 1984, c.6, s.1., Section 12 (1).
5. Lee Soderstrom, *The Canadian Health System* (London: Croom Helm, 1978), pp. 25–26.
6. Organisation for Economic Co-operation and Development, *OECD Health Systems, Facts and Trends 1960–1991,* Vol. 1 (Paris: OECD, 1993), table 5.2.7.
7. Cyril Nair, Rezaul Karim, and Christina Nyers, "Health Care and Health Status: A Canada–United States Statistical Comparison" *Health Reports* 4:2 (1992), p. 176.
8. W. Pete Welsh et al, "A Detailed Comparison of Physician Services for the Elderly in the United States and Canada," *Journal of the American Medical Association* 275:18 (May 8, 1996), pp. 1410–17.
9. Victor R. Fuchs and James S. Hahn, "How Does Canada Do It? A Comparison of Expenditures for Physicians' Services in the United States and Canada," *New England Journal of Medicine* 323:13 (Sept. 27, 1990), pp. 884–90.
10. Nair et al, "Health Care and Health Status," p. 180.
11. See Leah Beth Ward, "Heartening Signs for Specialty M.D.s," *New York Times* (Aug. 4, 1994), p. 8.
12. See Kassler, *Bitter Medicine,* p. 42.
13. Enterline et al, "Effects of 'Free' Medical Care," p. 285.
14. According to one recent study, while 97 percent of the residents of the more urbanized areas in Canada (those with 50,000 or more people) lived less than about three miles from the nearest doctor, only 67 percent of those in the less urban and rural areas did so. Edward Ng et al, "How Far to the Nearest Physician?" *Health Reports* 8:4 (spring 1997), table A.
15. Quoted in Ward, "Heartening Signs."
16. Nair et al, "Health Care and Health Status," p. 178.
17. Nair et al, "Health Care and Health Status," p. 178.
18. David U. Himmelstein, James P. Lewontin, and Steffie Woolhandler, "Who Administers? Who Cares? Medical Administrative and Clinical Employment in the United States and Canada," *American Journal of Public Health* 86:2 (Feb. 1996), table 2.
19. Statistics Canada, *Residential Care Facilities—Aged 1990–91* (Ottawa: Minister of Industry, Science and Technology, 1993), table 3.

20. OECD, *OECD Health Systems, Facts and Trends,* Table 5.2.4.

21. Statistics Canada, *Residential Care Facilities 1993,* cat. no. 83-240 (Ottawa: Minister of Industry, Science and Technology, 1994), table 1.

22. W. Pete Welch et al, "A Detailed Comparison of Physician Services," p. 1410.

23. Blair Richardson, "Overview of Provincial Homecare Programs in Canada," *Healthcare Management Forum* 3:3 (1990), pp. 3–10.

24. For a summary of the research, see Ann Crichton et al, *Health Care A Community Concern? Developments in the Organization of Canadian Health Services* (Calgary: University of Calgary Press, 1997), chapter 13.

25. Jonathan Lomas, *First and Foremost in Community Health Centres: The Centre at Sault Ste Marie and the CHC Alternative* (Toronto: University of Toronto Press, 1985), p. 71.

26. Quoted in Anne Crichton, Ann Robertson, Christine Gordon, Wendy Ferrant, *Health Care: A Community Concern.* Calgary: University of Calgary Press, p. 101.

27. A. Paul Williams et al, "A Typology of Medical Practice Organization in Canada," *Medical Care* 28:11 (1990), p. 996.

28. Robert Evans et al, "Who Are the Zombies' Masters, and What Do They Want?" (Toronto: Premier's Council on Health, Well-being and Social Justice, 1994), p. 3.

29. Morris Barer et al, "The Remarkable Tenacity of User Charges: A Concise History of the Participation, Positions, and Rationales of Canadian Interest Groups in the Debate Over 'Direct Patient Participation' in Health Care Financing" (Toronto: Premier's Council on Health, Well-being and Social Justice, 1994), p. 8 (emphasis in original).

30. Barer et al, "The Remarkable Tenacity," p. 27.

31. Cited in Greg Stoddart et al, "User Charges, Snares and Delusions: Another Look at the Literature" (Toronto: Premier's Council on Health, Well-being and Social Justice, 1994), p. 25.

32. Cited in Greg Stoddart et al, "Why Not User Charges? The Real Issues" (Toronto: Premier's Council on Health, Well-being and Social Justice, 1993), p. 7.

33. Cited in Stoddart et al, "Why Not User Charges?" p. 8.

34. See Robert G. Evans, *Strained Mercy: The Economics of Canadian Health Care* (Toronto: Butterworths, 1984), p. 333.

35. Quoted in Evans et al, "Who Are the Zombie Masters?," p. 11.

36. "Medicare Deductible, Coinsurance and Premium Amounts," *The Federal Register* vol. 61, no. 214, pages 55002–55009, October 23, 1996.

149

37. Jorge Segovia et al, "Medical Care Utilization: Policy Implications," a paper presented to the Seventh Canadian Conference on Health Economics, Ottawa, August 1997. Quoted with permission.

38. David U. Himmelstein and Steffie Woolhandler, *The National Health Program Book* (Monroe, ME: Common Courage Press, 1994), p. 94.

39. Milan Korcok, "CMPA Not Alone in Pursuing High Reserves, CMA's Survey of U.S. Firms Reveals," *Canadian Medical Association Journal* 154:12 (June 15, 1996), pp. 1891–94.

40. Maine People's Alliance, "The Litigation Explosion is a Myth," http://www.biddeford.com/mpa/medmal2.htm, p. 1 of 2, Mar. 7, 1997.

41. Statistics Canada, 1991 Census, *Employment Income By Occupation,* cat. no. 93-332 (Ottawa: Ministry of Industry, Science and Technology, 1993), table 1.

42. Cited in Jeanne Kassler, *Bitter Medicine* (New York: Birch Lane Press, 1994), p. 42.

43. Dr. Harrison's account is drawn from Elaine Medline, "Money Gives Doctors a Real Pain," *Ottawa Citizen* (Oct. 15, 1996), p. A4.

44. U.S. Bureau of Labor Statistics, *Employment and Wages, Annual Averages,* table 39, (ftp://stats. 1996). Lawrence C. Baker, "Differences in Earnings Between Male and Female Physicians," *New England Journal of Medicine* 334:15 (April 11, 1996), pp. 960–64.

45. Statistics Canada, *Employment Income by Occupation, Census 91* (Ottawa: Minister of Industry, Science and Technology, 1993), table 1; and OECD, *OECD Health Systems, Facts and Trends, 1960–91,* table 5.1.3.

46. Jennifer S. Haas and Lee Goldman, "Acutely Injured Patients With Trauma in Massachusetts: Differences in Care and Mortality, by Insurance Status," *American Journal of Public Health* 84:10 (Oct. 1994), p. 1605.

47. Peter C. Coyle et al, "Waiting Times for Knee-Replacement Surgery in the United States and Canada," *New England Journal of Medicine* 331:16 (Oct. 20, 1994), pp. 1068–71.

48. See Peggy Leatt and A. Paul Williams, "Canada," pp. 1–28 in Marshall W. Raffel, ed., *Health Care Reform in Industrialized Countries* (University Park, PA: The Pennsylvania State University Press, 1997), p. 15.

49. Steffie Woolhandler, Grand Rounds Presentations, February 1996, Department of Anesthesiology, Boston Children's Hospital, unpaginated table taken from Steffie Woolhandler and David U. Himmelstein, *The Case for Single Payer Reform,* The National Health Program Chartbook and

Slideshow, 1996 edition. The Center for National Health Program Studies, Harvard Medical School, Cambridge Hospital, 1996.

50. U.S. Census Bureau, "Health Insurance Coverage: 1995. Who Goes Without Coverage," http://www.census.gov/ffp/pub/hhes/hlthins/cover95asc.html, July 20, 1997, p. 1 of 3.

51. B. Singh Bolaria and Rosemary Bolaria, eds., *Racial Minorities in Medicine and Health* (Halifax: Fernwood, 1994).

52. National Forum on Health, "The Need for An Aboriginal Health Institute in Canada" *Canada Health Action: Building on the Legacy*, Vol. II, *Synthesis Reports and Issues Papers* (Ottawa: Minister of Public Works and Government Services, 1997).

53. Patricia Tulley and Chris Mohl, "Older Residents of Health Care Institutions," *Health Reports* 7:3 (1995), p. 27.

54. Alan Detsky, "Northern Exposure—Can the United States Learn from Canada?" *New England Journal of Medicine* 328:11 (Mar. 18, 1993), p. 805.

55. Pat Armstrong, "Women and Health: Challenges and Changes," in Nancy Mandell, ed., *Feminist Issues: Race, Class and Sexuality* (Scarborough: Prentice-Hall, 1995), pp. 294–314; National Forum on Health, "An Overview of Women's Health," *Canada Health Action: Building on the Legacy*, Vol. II, *Synthesis Reports and Issue Papers* (Ottawa: Minister of Public Works and Government Services, 1997).

56. National Forum on Health, "An Overview of Women's Health," p. 15.

57. Detsky, "Northern Exposure," p. 805.

CHAPTER 4. COMPREHENSIVE COVERAGE

1. Canada Health Act, Section 9.

2. Canada Health Act, Section 2.

3. Judy Haiven, "MediScare," *Mother Jones* (Mar.–Apr. 1991), p. 52.

4. Haiven, "MediScare," p. 52.

5. National Forum on Health, "Striking a Balance Working Group Synthesis Report," *Canada Health Action: Building on the Legacy*, Vol. II, *Synthesis Reports and Issues Papers* (Ottawa: Minister of Public Works and Government Services, 1997), p. 42; citing Jeremiah Hurley et al, "Defying Definition: Medical Necessity and Health Policy Making," Working Paper 96–15, Centre for Health Economics and Policy Analysis, McMaster University, Hamilton (August 1996).

6. Stephen M. Ayres, *Health Care in the United States: The Facts and The Choices* (Chicago: American Library Association, 1996), p. 17.
7. Monique Bégin, *Medicare: Canada's Right to Health*, Trans. by David Homel and Lucille Nelson (Montreal: Optimum Publishing, 1988), p. 173.
8. Canada Health Act, Section 2.
9. Health Canada, "National Health Expenditures in Canada 1975–1996: Fact Sheets" (Ottawa: Minister of Public Works and Government Services, 1997), table 4.
10. Health Canada, *National Health Expenditures*, table 4. These amounts are expressed in current Canadian dollars. If the effects of inflation are eliminated, the increase is of course less, but still remains relatively high at just over 100 percent over 21 years, compared to a 32 percent increase in real per capita spending on doctors (and a 17 percent increase in spending on hospitals) during this period. Calculated from *National Health Expenditures*, table 5.
11. See table 4.1. For another estimate, see National Forum on Health, "Directions for a Pharmaceutical Policy in Canada," *Canada Health Action: Building on the Legacy*, Vol. II, *Synthesis Reports and Issues Papers* (Ottawa: Minister of Public Works and Government Services, 1997), p. 3.
12. National Forum on Health, "Directions for a Pharmaceutical Policy," p. 4.
13. Joel Lexchin, "Income Class and Pharmaceutical Expenditures in Canada: 1964–1990," *Canadian Journal of Public Health* 87:1 (1996), pp. 46–50; and Joel Lexchin, *The Real Pushers* (Vancouver: New Star Books, 1984), p. 39.
14. National Forum on Health, "Discussions for a Pharmaceutical Policy," p. 4.
15. Lexchin, *The Real Pushers*, pp. 39–41.
16. See Benoit Champeaux, *An Economic Impact Analysis of the Retroactive Elimination of Compulsory Licensing*, Pharmaceutical Policy Division, Drugs Directorate, Health Protection Branch, Health Canada, 1995.
17. Michael Fitz-James, "Happy Birthday, Reference Based Pricing" *Canadian Healthcare Manager* (Oct.–Nov., 1996), pp. 12–17.
18. Fitz-James, "Happy Birthday," p. 12.
19. Fitz-James, "Happy Birthday," p. 13.
20. Organisation for Economic Co-operation and Development (OECD), "OECD Health Data 97," http://www.oecd.org/statlist.htm (updated July 8, 1997), Health II table.

21. OECD, "Health Data, 1993."

22. Cyril Nair and Rezaul Karim, "An Overview of Health Care Systems: Canada and Selected OECD Countries," *Health Reports* 5:3 (1993), table 5.

23. "OECD Health Data 97," Health II table.

24. Organisation for Economic Co-operation and Development, *OECD Health Systems: Facts and Trends 1960–1991* (Paris: OECD, 1993), table 3.1.9. The figures for Canada are from 1978 while those for the United States are from 1980. This is thus likely to underestimate rather than over-estimate the differences between the two countries in disability free years.

25. David U. Himmelstein and Steffie Woolhandler, *The National Health Program Book* (Monroe, ME: Common Courage Press, 1994), p. 145.

26. OECD, *OECD Health Systems,* table 3.2.4.

27. In Canada, the Canadian Council on Health Services Accreditation assures hospital standards. Across the border, this is done by the U.S. Joint Committee on Accreditation of Health Care Organizations.

28. Ronald A. Redelmeier and Victor R. Fuchs, "Hospital Expenditures in the United States and Canada," *New England Journal of Medicine* 328:11 (Mar. 18, 1993), p. 776.

29. David U. Himmelstein, James P. Lewontin, and Steffie Woolhandler, "Who Administers? Who Cares? Medical Administrative and Clinical Employment in the United States and Canada," *American Journal of Public Health* 86:2 (Feb. 1996), pp. 172–78. Calculated from table 2.

30. Himmelstein et al, "Who Administers?," p. 172.

31. Nair and Karem, "An Overview of Health Care Systems," table 3.

32. Jean L. Rouleau et al, "A Comparison of Management Patterns After Acute Myocardial Infarction in Canada and the United States," *New England Journal of Medicine* 328:11 (March 18, 1993), pp. 779–84.

33. OECD, *OECD Health Systems,* table 3.2.13.

34. Leslie L. Roos et al, "Health and Surgical Outcomes in Canada and the United States," *Health Affairs* 11:2 (Summer 1992), pp. 56–71.

35. Robert J. Blendon and Humphrey Taylor, "Views on Health Care: Public Opinion in Three Nations," *Health Affairs* (spring 1992), exhibit 3.

36. See Marshall W. Raffel, ed., *Health Care and Reform in Industrialized Countries* (University Park, Penn.: Pennsylvania State University Press, 1997). An article on Canada by Peggy Leatt and A. Paul Williams and one on the United States by Marshall W. Raffel and Norma K. Raffel summarize the accreditation processes in these countries.

37. Raffel and Raffel, in *Health Care and Reform,* p. 267.
38. Milan Korcok, "Medical-Management Guidelines Being Developed With a Vengeance in the US," *Canadian Medical Association Journal* 151:11 (Dec. 1, 1994), pp. 1625–27. For a brief description of the Milliman and Robertson guidelines, see Allen R. Myerson, "Helping Health Insurers Say No," *New York Times* (Mar. 20, 1995), pp. D1, D5.
39. Bob Carty, HMO documentary, *Sunday Morning,* CBS radio, Sunday, January 12, 1997.
40. Carty, HMO documentary.
41. Milan Korcok, "Medical Management Guidelines," p. 1627.
42. Elizabeth A. McGlynn et al, "Comparisons of the Appropriateness of Coronary Angiography and Coronary Heart Bypass Graft Surgery Between Canada and New York State," *Journal of the American Medical Association* 272:12 (Sept. 28, 1994), pp. 934–37.
43. Louise Pilote, Normand Racine, and Mark A. Hlatky, "Differences in the Treatment of Myocardial Infarction in the United States and Canada: Comparison of Two University Hospitals," *Archives of Internal Medicine* 154:10 (May 23, 1994), pp. 1090–97.
44. Rouleau et al, "A Comparison of Management Patterns," pp. 779–84.
45. Blendon and Taylor, "Views On Health Care," exhibit 6.
46. *Health Progress* (Jan.–Feb. 1994).
47. David Feeny, "Technology Assessment and Health Policy in Canada," pp. 275–326 in Ake Blomquist and David M. Brown, eds., *Limits to Care: Reforming Canada's Health System in an Age of Restraint* (Toronto: C. D. Howe Institute, 1994).
48. Feeny, "Technology Assessment," p. 302.
49. *Health Progress.*
50. Harlan Krumholz, "Cardiac Procedures, Outcomes and Accountability," *New England Journal of Medicine* 336:21 (May 22, 1997), p. 1522.

CHAPTER 5. PORTABILITY:
YOU *CAN* TAKE IT WITH YOU

1. Jerome P. Kassirer, "Access to Specialty Care," *New England Journal of Medicine* 331:17 (Oct. 27, 1994), pp. 1151–53.
2. Air Ambulance Review Committee (G. L. Donner, chair), *Final Report* (Toronto: Queen's Printer for Ontario, 1994), pp. iii, 13.
3. Cited in Allan S. Detsky, "Northern Exposure—Can the United States

154

Learn from Canada?" *New England Journal of Medicine* 328:11 (Mar. 18, 1993), p. 805; and in John K. Inglehart, "The American Health Care System—Introduction," *New England Journal of Medicine* 326:14 (Apr. 2, 1992), p. 962, respectively.

4. Kassirer, "Access to Specialty Care," p. 1151.
5. Canada Health Act, 1984, 11(1)(6).
6. Canada Health Act, 1984, 11(2).
7. Canada Health Act, 1984, 11(3).
8. Canada Health Act, 1984, 11(2).
9. Detsky, "Northern Exposure," p. 806.

CHAPTER 6. PUBLIC ADMINISTRATION

1. Canada Health Act, 8(1)(a).
2. Charles P. Schade, "A Preliminary Comparison Between Local Public Health Units in the Canadian Province of Ontario and the United States," *Public Health Reports* 110:1 (January–February 1995), pp. 35–37.
3. Marc Lalonde, *A New Perspective on Health For Canadians* (Ottawa: Supply and Services Canada, 1974); Jake Epp, *Achieving Health for All: A Framework for Health Promotion* (Ottawa: Supply and Services Canada, 1986).
4. Ann Pederson, Michel O'Neill, and Irving Rootman, eds., *Health Promotion in Canada: Provincial, National and International Perspectives* (Toronto: W. B. Saunders, 1994).
5. See Statistics Canada, *Hospital Annual Statistics: 1994–95,* cat. no. 82-241 (Ottawa: Ministry of Industry, Science and Technology, 1996); and Pat Armstrong and Hugh Armstrong, *Wasting Away: The Undermining of Canadian Health Care* (Toronto: Oxford University Press, 1996).
6. Statistics Canada, *List of Residential Care Facilities,* cat. no. 83-240 (Ottawa: Ministry of Industry, Science and Technology, 1994), table 1.
7. Organisation for Economic Co-operation and Development, "OECD Health Data 97." http://www.oecd.org/statlist.htm (updated July 8, 1997), Health II table.
8. U.S. Census Bureau, *Health Insurance Coverage, 1995. Highlights* (Washington: U.S. Census Bureau, 1996).
9. Canada, Department of Foreign Affairs and International Trade. "Overview of Taxation in Canada, the United States and Mexico," World Wide Web, Aug. 8, 1997.

10. Canadian Centre for Policy Alternatives, *CCPA Monitor,* "Canada's Payroll Taxes Lowest of All G7 Countries" (February 1997), p. 24.

11. KPMG Canada, "Benefit Cost Survey," World Wide Web, August 8, 1997, http://ns.kpmg.ca/hr/surveys/hr-bnfit.htm.

12. David U. Himmelstein and Steffie Woolhandler, *The National Health Program Book* (Monroe, ME: Common Courage Press, 1994), p. 41.

13. Himmelstein and Woolhandler, *National Health Program Book,* p. 176.

14. Health Canada, "National Health Expenditures in Canada, 1975–1996: Fact Sheets" (Ottawa: Minister of Public Works and Government Services, 1997), calculated from table 2.

15. Stephen M. Ayres, *Health Care in the United States: The Facts and the Choices* (Chicago: American Library Association, 1996), Fig. 1–3.

16. Health Canada, *National Health Expenditures in Canada 1975–1994: Full Report* (Ottawa: Supply and Services Canada, 1996), pp. 22–23.

17. Donald A. Redelmeier and Victor Fuchs, "Hospital Expenditures in the United States and Canada," *New England Journal of Medicine* 328:11 (Mar. 18, 1993), p. 776.

18. David U. Himmelstein, James P. Lewontin, and Steffie Woolhandler, "Who Administers? Who Cares? Medical Administrative and Clinical Employment in the United States and Canada," *American Journal of Public Health* 86:2 (Feb. 1996), pp. 172–78.

19. Himmelstein et al, "Who Administers?" p. 175.

20. According to one estimate, U.S. doctors together spent $US 330 per capita on billing and office expenses in 1993, or over 2.3 times the $US 142 spent by Canadian doctors. Himmelstein and Woolhandler, *National Health Program Book,* p. 134.

21. Murray Mandryk, "Doctor Moves Back from the U.S.," *Regina Leader Post* (Jan. 18, 1997), quoting Dr. Volker Rininsland.

22. Jerome P. Kassirer, "Managing Managed Care's Tarnished Image," *New England Journal of Medicine* 337:5 (July 31, 1997), p. 339.

23. FamiliesUSA, "Consumer Concerns about Managed Care Spur Avalanche of State Legislative Action," press release dated July 23, 1996, on the occasion of the publication of its report entitled "HMO Consumers at Risk: States to the Rescue." FamiliesUSA describes itself as "the national nonprofit organization for health care consumers" and can be reached by phone at (202) 628-3030.

24. Canada Health Act, Section 8.

25. National Forum on Health, "Striking a Balance Working Group Synthesis Report," *Canada Health Action: Building on the Legacy,* Vol. II, *Synthesis Reports and Issues Papers,* (Ottawa: Minister of Public Works and Government Services, 1997), p. 16.

26. Jeanne Kassler, *Bitter Medicine: Greed and Chaos in American Health Care* (New York: Birch Lane Press, 1994), p. xii.

27. "Mercky Waters," *The Economist* (May 24, 1997), p. 59.

28. Frank Cerne, "Cash Kings," *Hospitals and Health Networks* (Apr. 5, 1995), p. 52, reporting on a study by Volpe, Welty & Co.

29. Physicians for a National Health Program (PNHP), *Newsletter* (Nov. 1996), p. 5, citing *Jenks Healthcare Business Report* (Sept. 24, 1996).

30. Michael A. Hiltzik and David R. Olmos, "Are Executives at HMOs Paid Too Much Money?" *Los Angeles Times* (Aug. 30, 1995).

31. PNHP, *Newsletter* (Nov. 1996), p. 5, citing *New York Times* (June 15, 1996).

32. Milt Freudenheim, "Cigna to Buy Healthsource, Vaulting Ahead in H.M.O.'s," *New York Times* (Mar. 1, 1997), p. 37.

33. Fred Schulte and Jenni Bergal, "HMO's Profits, Complaints Piled Up," reprint from the "Profits from Pain" series, *Fort Lauderdale Sun-Sentinel* (Dec. 11–15, 1994), p. 5. In 1991, Better Health Plan had revenues of $38 million, all from the state's publicly funded Medicare program, and paid out 19 percent of this total in salaries to its three owners.

34. Himmelstein and Woolhandler, *National Health Program Book,* p. 48.

35. Ayres, *Health Care in the United States,* pp. 17–18.

36. Himmelstein and Woolhandler, *National Health Program Book,* p. 126.

37. Ed Cooper and Liz Taylor, "Comparing Health Care Systems," *In Context* 39 (fall 1994), p. 36.

38. Redelmeier and Fuchs, "Hospital Expenditures," p. 777.

39. Canadian Health Coalition, advertisement in *The Hill Times* (Jan. 20, 1997), p. 13.

40. Patrick Sullivan, "CMA Calls for Controls on Prescription-Drug Advertising Aimed at Patients," *Canadian Medical Association Journal* 154:12 (June 15, 1996), pp. 1889–90.

41. National Forum on Health, "Directions for a Pharmaceutical Policy in Canada," *Canada Health Action: Building on the Legacy,* Vol. II, *Synthesis Reports and Issues Papers,* (Ottawa: Minister of Public Works and Government Services, 1996), pp. 4–5.

42. See for example Nancy Watzman and Patrick Woodall, "Managed Care Companies' Lobbying Frenzy," and The Center for Public Integrity, "Well-Healed: Inside Lobbying for Health Care Reform," *International Journal of Health Services* 25:3 (1995), pp. 403–10 and 411–53, respectively. Another reason is that the congressional system of government provides more scope for lobbying than does the parliamentary system with its tighter party discipline. Even among the parliamentary democracies, Canada is known to have particularly tight party discipline.

43. C. David Naylor, "A Different View of Queues in Ontario," *Health Affairs* (fall 1991), pp. 111–28.

44. Naylor, "A Different View," p. 116.

45. Naylor, "A Different View," p. 111.

46. PNHP, *Newsletter,* citing a KPMG survey.

CHAPTER 7. A PERFECT SYSTEM?

1. H. Mimoto and P. Cross, "The Growth of the Federal Debt," *Canadian Economic Observer* (June 1991), pp. 1–17.

2. World Economic Forum, *World Competitiveness Report 1991* (Lausanne, Switzerland: Institut pour l'étude des méthodes de direction de l'entreprise, 1992).

3. Tom Closson and Margaret Catt, "Funding System Incentives and the Restructuring of Health Care," *Canadian Journal of Public Health* 87:2 (March–April 1996), Table IV.

4. Reported in Robert Pear, "Health Costs Pose Problems for Millions, A Study Finds," *New York Times* (October 23, 1996), p. A4.

5. National Forum on Health, "Striking a Balance Working Group Synthesis Report," *Canada Health Action: Building on the Legacy,* Vol. II, *Synthesis Reports and Issues Papers* (Ottawa: Minister of Public Works and Government Services, 1997), p. 39.

6. Miro Cernetig and Robert Matas, "B.C. Can't Limit Where MDs Set Up Practices, Court Rules," Toronto *Globe and Mail* (Aug. 2, 1997), pp. A1, A7. Contrast this situation to that in the United States where, according to a recent report, at least 5 percent of new graduates in eleven of twenty-four specialties cannot find full-time positions anywhere, and "most job offers come from far-flung places, not urban areas." Leah Beth Ward, "Heartening Signs for Specialty M.D.'s," *New York Times* (Aug. 4, 1996),

p. F8, reporting on a study in a March 1996 issue of the *Journal of the American Medical Association*.

7. Between 75 and 80 percent of registered nurses employed in the Canadian health care system are unionized, as against between 10 and 15 percent in the United States. Kit Costello, "Canadian Nurses—Our Northern Neighbors Fight Similar Battles," *California Nurse* 93:6 (June–July 1997), p. 12. Salaries for Canadian nurses averaged $US 39,161 for 37.5 hours work a week in 1992, as against $34,192 for 39.5 hours in the United States. Judith Shindul-Rothschild and Suzanne Gordon, "Single-Payer Versus Managed Competition: Implications for Nurses," *Journal of Nursing Education* 33:5 (May 1994), p. 204.

8. Greg L. Stoddart et al, "Why Not User Charges? The Real Issues," a discussion paper prepared for the [Ontario] Premier's Council on Health, Well-being and Social Justice (Sept. 1993), pp. 5–6.

9. Stoddart et al, "Why Not User Charges?," p. 5 (emphasis in original).

10. Jane Coutts, "Medicare Gives Poor a Better Chance," Toronto *Globe and Mail* (Aug. 1, 1997), p. A1.

11. See National Forum on Health, "Creating a Culture of Evidence-Based Decision-Making," *Canada Health Action: Building on the Legacy,* Vol. II, *Synthesis Reports and Issues Papers* (Ottawa: Minister of Public Works and Government Services, 1997), esp. pp. 21–23.

12. David U. Himmelstein and Steffie Woolhandler, *The National Health Program Book* (Monroe, ME: Common Courage Press, 1994), p. 109. In 1990, the U.S. figure was 526 articles per million population, while the Canadian figure was 520. Both were well behind Israel, Sweden, and the United Kingdom, but well ahead of Germany and Japan.

13. Noralou P. Roos et al, "Population Health and Health Care Use: An Information System for Policy Makers," *Milbank Quarterly* 74:1 (spring 1996), pp. 3–31.

14. Health Canada, "National Health Expenditures in Canada 1975–1996: Fact Sheets," (Ottawa: Minister of Public Works and Government Services, 1997), tables 4 and 5. The percentage increase is presented "in real terms" in order to eliminate the impact of inflation.

15. Michael Fitz-James, "Happy Birthday, Reference-Based Pricing," *Canadian Healthcare Manager* 3:6 (Oct.–Nov. 1996), p. 12.

16. *Report* of the [Eastman] Commission of Inquiry on the Pharmaceutical Industry (Ottawa: Supply and Services Canada, 1985).

17. National Forum on Health, "Directions for a Pharmaceutical Policy in

Canada," *Canada Health Action: Building on the Legacy,* Vol. II, *Synthesis Reports and Issues Papers* (Ottawa: Minister of Public Works and Government Services, 1997), p. 5.

18. See for example R. B. Coambes et al, *Review of the Literature on the Prevalence, Consequences, and Health Costs of Noncompliance and Inappropriate Use of Prescription Medication in Canada.* Prepared for the Pharmaceutical Manufacturers Association of Canada. (Toronto: University of Toronto Press, 1995); Joel Lexchin, "Canadian Marketing Codes: How Well Are They Controlling Pharmaceutical Promotion?" *International Journal of Health Services* 24:1 (1996); Joel Lexchin, *The Real Pushers: A Critical Analysis of the Canadian Drug Industry* (Vancouver: New Star Books, 1984).

19. National Forum on Health, "Directions for a Pharmaceutical Policy," p. 18.

20. Charles J. Wright, "Physician Remuneration: Fee-for-service Must Go, But Then What?," pp. 35–38 in Raisa B. Deber and Gail G. Thompson, eds., *Restructuring Canada's Health Service System: How Do We Get There from Here?* (Toronto: University of Toronto Press, 1992).

21. Ann Crichton et al, *Health Care A Community Concern? Developments in the Organization of Canadian Health Services* (Calgary: University of Calgary Press, 1997).

22. Thomas S. Bodenheimer and Kevin Grumbach, "Capitation or Decapitation: Keeping Your Head in Changing Times," *Journal of the American Medical Association* 276:13 (Oct. 2, 1996), pp. 1025–31. See also Pat Armstrong, "Managing the Canadian Way," *Humane Health Care International* (formerly *Humane Medicine*) 13:1 (spring 1997), pp. 13–14.

23. Organisation for Economic Co-operation and Development, *Health Care Reform: The Will to Change* (Paris: OECD, 1996).

24. Among the reasons why health care cannot be transformed into an efficient market are these. The services are often required on an urgent or emergency basis, which is no time for comparative shopping. The consequences of bad choices can be literally fatal. The consumers, or patients, typically lack sufficient knowledge with which to make informed choices on complex matters, which is in turn one reason why many who work in health care are accorded the status and responsibility of being considered "professionals." The complexity of health care and the interdependence of its many components, involving different skills among a wide range of providers and expensive facilities such as hospitals, mean that integrated care could be purchased from only a very few organizations. Each would

have to serve perhaps a quarter or half a million people, preventing competition in all but the largest cities. Finally, the trust that is required to make all the complex parts of health care mesh together takes years to build up and cannot be captured in contractual language. All these considerations apply to markets in both the public and private sectors. If the market is private and for-profit, there is of course the further problem that for-profit firms must seek to maximize profits, and do so in part by cutting the quality and quantity of what they produce.

25. In Canada as in the United States, this faith is often expressed as the need to "reinvent government" by having it set broad public policy objectives but turn the implementation of public policy over to the private sector through time-limited contracts. The term was popularized by David Osborne and Ted Gaebler in their widely cited book, *Reinventing Government: How the Entrepreneurial Spirit Is Transforming the Public Sector* (New York: Penguin, 1993).

26. Philip Hassen, *Rx for Hospitals: New Hope for Medicare in the Nineties* (Toronto: Stoddart, 1993), p. 63.

27. For an assessment of the effects of introducing TQM into hospital settings, see Pat Armstrong et al, "The Promise and the Price," pp. 31–68 in Pat Armstrong et al, *Medical Alert: New Work Organizations in Health Care* (Toronto: Garamond Press, 1997).

28. Working Group on Health Services Utilization, "When Less is Better: Using Canada's Hospitals Efficiently," a report to the Federal/Provincial/Territorial Deputy Ministers of Health (June 1994).

29. See Pat Armstrong, "Closer to Home: More Work for Women," pp. 95–110 in Pat Armstrong et al, *Take Care: Warning Signals for Canada's Health System* (Toronto: Garamond Press, 1994).

30. National Forum on Health, "Striking a Balance," p. 26.

31. Health Canada, "National Health Expenditures in Canada 1975–1996: Fact Sheets" (Ottawa: Minister of Public Works and Government Services, 1997), Table 2.

32. Jerome P. Kassirer, "Managing Managed Care's Tarnished Image," *New England Journal of Medicine* 337:5 (July 31, 1997), p. 338, citing L. Kertesz, "HMO Makeover," *Modern Healthcare* (May 12, 1997), pp. 36–46.

33. Health and Welfare Canada, *Privatization in the Canadian Health Care System: Assertions, Evidence, Ideology and Options* (Ottawa: Health and Welfare Canada, 1985), p. 68.

Further Reading

BOOKS AND ARTICLES

Pat Armstrong and Hugh Armstrong, in *Wasting Away: The Undermining of Canadian Health Care* (Toronto: Oxford University Press, 1996), describe the impact the current reforms are having on the Canadian health care system. In addition, Pat Armstrong has produced several edited books that bring together providers' views of health reform. These include: *Medical Alert: New Work Organizations in Health Care* (Toronto: Garamond Press, 1997) with Hugh Armstrong, Jacqueline Choiniere, Eric Mykhalovskiy, and Jerry P. White; *Take Care: Warning Signals for Canadian Health Care* (Toronto: Garamond Press, 1994) with Hugh Armstrong, Jacqueline Choiniere, Gina Feldberg, and Jerry White; and *Vital Signs: Nursing in Transition* (Toronto: Garamond Press, 1993) with Jacqueline Choiniere and Elaine Day.

Robert G. Evans, a well-known health economist, has produced several books that provide broad analyses of economic issues in health care. The first of these, *Strained Mercy: The Economics of Canadian Health Care* (Toronto: Butterworths, 1984) has become a classic text. *Medicare at Maturity: Achievements, Lessons and Challenges* (Calgary: University of Calgary Press, 1989), a book he co-edited with Greg L. Stoddart, takes up a series of issues related to the management of health care resources.

Excellent historical analyses of the development of health insurance in Canada can be found in: Malcolm Taylor, *Health Insurance and Ca-*

nadian Public Policy: The Seven Decisions That Created the Canadian Health Insurance System and Their Outcomes, 2nd ed. (Kingston and Montreal: McGill–Queen's University Press, 1987); and C. David Naylor, *Private Practice, Public Payment: Canadian Medicine and the Politics of Health Insurance 1911–1966* (Kingston and Montreal: McGill-Queen's University Press, 1986).

On the achievement of medical insurance in Saskatchewan, see Robin F. Badgley and Samuel Wolfe, *Doctor's Strike: Medical Care and Conflict in Saskatchewan* (Toronto: Macmillan, 1967). For an insider's account of the events surrounding the passage of the Canada Health Act, see Monique Bégin, *Medicare: Canada's Right to Health* David Homel and Lucille Nelson, trans. (Montreal: Optimum Publishing, 1988).

Compiled by Helen Heeney and edited by Susan Charters, *Life Before Medicare: Canadian Experiences* (Toronto: The Stories Project, 1995) offers vivid personal accounts of illness in Canada in the years prior to the introduction of public health insurance. The book is available from the Ontario Coalition of Senior Citizens Organizations, 25 Cecil Street, 3rd Floor, Toronto ON Canada M5T 1N1; Phone: (416)979–7057, Fax: (416)977–9591.

Canada has taken the lead in health promotion. Marc Lalonde's *A New Perspective on Health for Canadians* (Ottawa: Minister of Supply and Services, 1974) set the framework for international discussions. He was followed by another federal Minister of Health, Jake Epp, who released *Achieving Health for All: A Framework for Health Promotion* (Ottawa: Supply and Services Canada, 1986). Examples of current thinking on health promotion can be found in Ann Pederson, Michel O'Neill and Irving Rootman, ed., *Health Promotion in Canada: Provincial, National and International Perspectives* (Toronto: W. B. Saunders, 1994).

A variety of books have promoted reforms to the Canadian health system, reforms that maintain the single-payer, universal aspects of the plan while moving in new directions. Among these are two by Michael Rachlis and Carol Kushner, *Second Opinion: What's Wrong with Canada's Health System and How to Fix It* (Toronto: HarperCollins, 1989); and *Strong Medicine: How to Save Canada's Health System* (Toronto: HarperCollins, 1994). Many of the reforms currently being proposed and implemented are assessed in Raisa B. Deber and Gail G. Thompson, eds., *Restructuring Canada's Health Services System: How Do We Get There from Here?* (Toronto: University of Toronto Press, 1992); and in Douglas J. McCready and William R. Swan, eds., *Change & Resistance* (Kingston: Canadian Health Economics Research Association, 1997). An important article by Sharmila L. Mhatre and Raisa B. Deber, "From Equal Access to Health Care to Equitable Access to Health: A Review of Canadian Provincial Health Commissions and Reports," *International Journal of Health Services* 22:4(1992), pp. 645–68, sets out several themes that run through the reform activities.

Although most health care in Canada is delivered through hospitals and doctors' offices, a number of provinces have long-standing traditions of community clinics that are similar to the early nonprofit HMOs in the United States. Jonathan Lomas's *First and Foremost in Community Health Centres: The Centre in Sault Ste Marie and the CHC Alternative* (Toronto: University of Toronto Press, 1985) analyzes a center established in Ontario by the United Steelworkers of America during the 1950s. Saskatchewan has also experimented with community clinics, and Stan Rands offers an insider's view of their development in *Privilege and Policy: A History of Community Clinics in Saskatchewan* (Saskatoon: Community Health Cooperative Federation, 1994). The federation can be reached at 455 Second Avenue North, Saskatoon, Saskatchewan, Canada S7K 2C2.

The CLSCs (*centres locaux de services communitaires,* or local community service centres) in Quebec have received considerable attention as a provincial initiative designed to bring together doctors, nurses, social workers, and community organizers in primary care organizations to meet all the social and health needs of a specific population. See Fréderic Lesemann, *Services and Circuses: Community and the Welfare State* Lorne Huston and Margaret Heap trans. (Montreal: Black Rose Books, 1984), especially chapter 5; Marc Renaud, "Reform or Illusion: An Analysis of the Quebec State Intervention in Health," pp. 590–614 in David Coburn et al, eds., *Health and Canadian Society: Sociological Perspectives* 2nd ed. (Richmond Hill ON: Fitzhenry and Whiteside, 1987); and Michel O'Neill, "Community Participation in Quebec's Health System: A Strategy to Curtail Community Empowerment?" *International Journal of Health Services* 22:2 (1992), pp. 287–301. Community participation in aspects of health care is the central theme in another useful overview of Canadian developments in health care: Ann Crichton et al, *Health Care a Community Concern? Developments in the Organization of Canadian Health Service* (Calgary: University of Calgary Press, 1997).

GOVERNMENT DOCUMENTS

Health Canada's Policy and Consultation Branch has for several years produced useful reports on health spending, the most recent of which is "National Health Expenditures in Canada 1975–1996: Fact Sheets." This report is available on Health Canada's internet home page at http://www.hwc.ca/datacbhesa/hex.htm. For further information, contact the Branch at: Health Canada, Brooke Claxton Building, Tunney's Pasture, Ottawa, Canada K1A 0K9; Phone: (613) 957–3080, Fax: (613) 957–1204.

Information on health expenditures, along with other health information, is increasingly the responsibility of the Canadian Institute for Health Information, 377 Dalhousie Street, Suite 200, Ottawa, Canada K1N 9N8; Phone: (613) 241–7860, Fax: (613) 241–8120 website: http://www.cihi.ca.

In 1994, the Prime Minister of Canada appointed twenty-four individuals who were knowledgeable about health care issues to serve as volunteer members of an advisory body on the health system in Canada. This body, known as the National Forum on Health, reported in 1997. Its publications provide a synthesis of issues raised by both experts and ordinary citizens and a series of recommendations about the future of health care. The final report includes:

Canada Health Action: Building on the Legacy, Vol. I, *The Final Report of the National Forum on Health.*

Canada Health Action: Building on the Legacy, Vol. II, *Synthesis Reports and Issues Papers*

Values Working Group Synthesis Report
Determinants of Health Working Group Synthesis Report
Striking a Balance Working Group Synthesis Report
Creating a Culture of Evidence-Based Decision Making
The Need for an Aboriginal Health Institute in Canada
Directions for a Pharmaceutical Policy in Canada
An Overview of Women's Health

Earlier reports from the National Forum included:

Let's Talk . . . About Our Health and Health Care
Health and Health Care Issues
The Public and Private Financing of Health Care

A number of research papers commissioned by the Forum are also due to be published in the near future. Publications are available from: National Forum on Health, P.O. Box 2798, 4th Floor, 200 Kent Street, Ottawa, Canada K1P 6H4; website: http://wwwnfh.hwc.ca.

Statistics Canada. This federal agency collects data on a wide range of issues, including annual statistics on hospitals and residential care facilities. Statistics Canada can be called toll-free at 1 (800) 267–6677.

Canada often begins new policy development by first establishing a Royal Commission or Task Force to investigate the issue. Health care is no exception. Three federal investigations of central importance are: Canada, *Report of the Royal Commission on Health Services* [Hall Royal Commission] (Ottawa: Queen's Printer, 1964); Canada, Health and Welfare Canada, *Reports of the Task Force on the Costs of Health Services*, 3 vols. (Ottawa: Information Canada, 1970); and Canada, Health and Welfare Canada, *Canada's National–Provincial Health Program for the 1980s: A Commitment for Renewal* [Hall Report] (Ottawa: Health and Welfare Canada, 1980).

A Quebec Commission of Inquiry established in 1966 had a much broader mandate than the federal Hall Royal Commission. It studied all aspects of health and social welfare, and recommended an integrated approach to the full range of health and social services. Quebec, *Report of the Commission of Inquiry on Health and Social Services* [Castonguay-

Nepveu Commission], 7 vols. (Quebec: Gouvernement du Quebec, 1967–72). These volumes seem remarkably modern today, reflecting current views on the determinants of health, democratic control, and the integrated management of care.

The Ontario Premier's Council on Health, Well-being and Social Justice published a comprehensive and accessible series of reports evaluating the research on user fees, that is, on additional charges paid by those using the health care system. These include:

Greg L. Stoddart et al, "Why Not User Charges? The Real Issues" (September 1993)

Morris L. Barer et al, "The Remarkable Tenacity of User Charges: A Concise History of the Participation, Positions and Rationales of Canadian Interest Groups in the Debate over 'Direct Patient Participation' in Health Care Financing" (June 1994)

Robert G. Evans et al, "User Charges in Health Care: A Bibliography" (June 1994).

Robert G. Evans et al, "Who Are the Zombies, and What Do They Want?" (June 1994)

Robert G. Evans et al, "It's Not the Money, It's the Principle: Why User Charges for Some Services and Not Others?" (June 1994)

Robert G. Evans et al, "Charging Peter to Pay Paul: Accounting for the Financial Effects of User Charges" (June 1994)

Greg L. Stoddart et al, "User Charges, Snares and Delusions: Another Look at the Literature" (June 1994)

The Ontario Premier's Council has since been disbanded. Inquiries about these publications may be directed to Publications Ontario, 50 Grosvenor Street, Toronto ON Canada M7A 1N8; Phone: (416) 326–5300, Fax: (416) 326–5317.

RELEVANT LEGISLATION

Canada, Hospital Insurance and Diagnostic Services Act, 1957. Ch. 28. This act introduced the federal insurance plan for hospital services.

Canada, Health Resources Fund Act, 1966. Ch. 42. This act established a fund to assist provinces in building health training facilities and research institutions.

Canada, Medical Care Act, 1966. Ch. 64. This legislation provided for a funding system designed to develop universal insurance for medical practitioners, that is, for doctors.

Canada, Canada Health Act, 1984. Ch. C-6. The Canada Health Act brought together the hospital and medical insurance plans at the same time as it set out clear definitions of the five principles that are the central criteria for federal funding.

Canada, Federal–Provincial Fiscal Arrangements and Established Programs Financing Act, 1977. This legislation changed the funding formula for health care and post-secondary education. Instead of paying half the health care bills, the federal government began paying on a per capita basis with adjustments made to ensure inter-provincial equity.

Canada, Patent Act Amendment Act, 1992 [Bill C-91, which became law in 1993]. This act eliminated the compulsory licensing of patented drugs by generic drug manufacturers, and extended the brand name companies' monopoly to 20 years.

Canada, Budget Implementation Act, 1995. This act replaced previous legislation covering the financing of not only health and post-secondary education but also of social assistance. Federal funding for all three program fields was combined under the new Canada Health and Social Transfer (CHST).

INTERNATIONAL COMPARISONS

The Organisation for Economic Co-operation and Development (OECD) is an excellent source of comparative data on health systems in the twenty-odd Western countries that belong to the organisation. Particularly relevant are its Health Policy Studies, including the following publications: *OECD Health Systems: Facts and Trends 1960– 1991*, Vol. 1 (Paris: OECD, 1993); *OECD Health Systems: The Socio- economic Environment*, Vol. II, (Paris: OECD, 1993); *The Reform of Health Care Systems–A Review of Seventeen OECD Countries* (Paris: OECD, 1994); *Internal Markets in the Making—Health Systems in Canada, Iceland and the United Kingdom* (Paris: OECD, 1995); and *Health Care Reform: The Will to Change* (Paris: OECD, 1996).

Marshall W. Raffel (ed.), *Health Care and Reform in Industrialized Countries* (University Park, PA: The Pennsylvania State University Press, 1997), is a book offering concise summaries of the major aspects of health systems in ten Western countries, including Canada and the United States. David U. Himmelstein and Steffie Woolhandler, in *The National Health Program Book* (Monroe ME: Common Courage Press, 1994), compare the Canadian and U.S. systems in a variety of ways, especially in parts V, VI and VIII.

Index